The
Shoulder Patients' Handbook

Disclaimer
This book is an educational resource to provide general information on shoulder injuries and treatments.
It is not intended to treat, diagnose or prescribe. It in no way is a substitute for the recommendations or
treatment of a licensed health care professional.

Cover design: Rob Diebold, Design Sonoma

Illustrations by: Denise Thompson

ISBN: 1439270600
EAN-13: 9781439270608

The
Shoulder Patients' Handbook

A Shoulder Surgeon's guide to Rotator Cuff Injuries and other common shoulder problems

PAUL B. ROACHE, MD

About the Author

Paul B. Roache, MD
Shoulder and Sports Medicine Specialist

Practice Focus

Dr. Roache is board certified by the American Board of Orthopedic Surgeons and is a fellow in the American Academy of Orthopaedic Surgeons. He is an associate member of the Arthroscopic Association of North America and is fellowship trained in shoulder and upper extremity surgery.

Dr. Roache's main subspecialty focus is in arthroscopic treatments of rotator cuff disorders, frozen shoulder, and shoulder dislocations. In addition, he has strong specialty interest in the arthroscopic treatment of sports medicine injuries to the knee. His main practice is in San Francisco. He is also a visiting attending surgeon during ski season at Mt. Crested Butte Ski Clinic in Colorado.

Recently, Dr. Roache has developed an interest in yoga as it relates to orthopaedic injuries. He is currently working with local yoga teachers and their students to develop techniques for injury identification and practice modifications to prevent further injury. He is a certified yoga teacher.

Education History:

St. Ignatius College Preparatory, San Francisco, CA
University of California Berkeley, Berkeley, CA
Loyola Marymount University, Los Angeles, CA

Medical Training:

University of Arizona, College of Medicine, Tucson, AZ
Internship: Santa Clara Valley Medical Center, San Jose, CA
Trauma Fellowship: Boston City Hospital, Boston, MA
Orthopaedic Residency: Albert Einstein College of Medicine, Bronx, NY
Shoulder Fellowship: California Pacific Medical Center, San Francisco, CA
AO Shoulder Fellowship: University of Balgrist, Zurich, Switzerland

Personal

Dr. Roache is a native of San Francisco and currently lives in San Francisco. He enjoys swimming, yoga, scuba diving, salsa dancing and skiing.

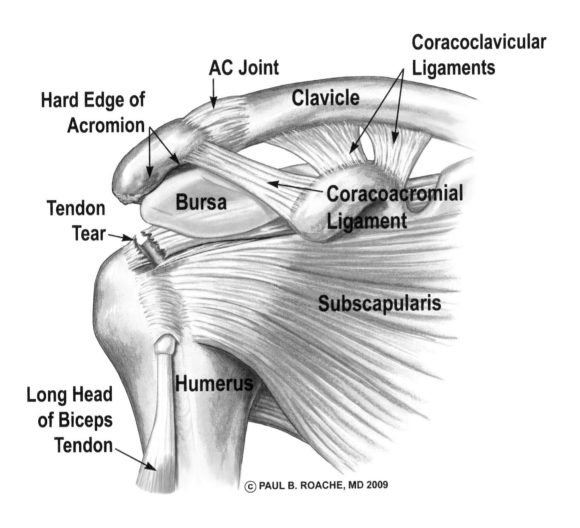

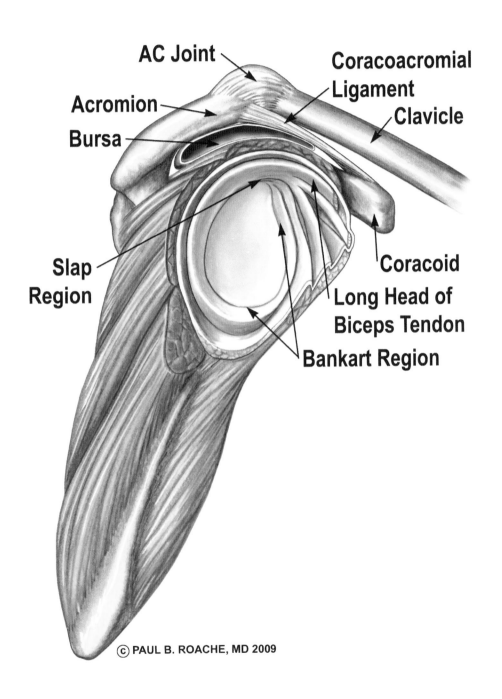

AC Joint

Acromion

Bursa

Slap
Region

Coracoacromial
Ligament

Clavicle

Coracoid

Long Head of
Biceps Tendon

Bankart Region

© PAUL B. ROACHE, MD 2009

☤ <u>Your diagnosis:</u>

○ Right Shoulder

○ Left Shoulder

❑ Rotator Cuff tear: *(see chapters 1,2 & 3)*

    ○ Partial thickness of the tendon

    ○ Fully torn

❑ Subacromial Impingement (pinching of the Bursa and cuff):
                                                      (see chapters 1,2 & 3)

    ○ With bone spur

    ○ Without bone spur

    ○ With AC joint arthritis/inflammation

❑ Instability/ Dislocation: *(see chapters 1 & 8)*

    ○ Anterior tear of labrum and ligament (Bankart)

    ○ Posterior tear of labrum

    ○ Multiple Directions/ligament laxity

❑ SLAP Tear: *(see chapters 1 & 9)*

    ○ Partial (Type 1)

    ○ Complete (Type 2)

❑ Biceps Tear/ Injury: *(see chapters 1 & 9)*

❑ Adhesive Capsulitis/ Frozen Shoulder: *(see chapters 1, 6 & 7)*

❑ AC Joint Injury: *(see chapters 1 & 12)*

❑ Fracture of the Clavicle: *(see chapters 1 & 11)*

❑ Fracture of the Proximal Humerus: *(see chapters 1 & 13)*

❑ Arthritis of the Glenohumeral Joint: *(see chapters 1 & 14)*

⚕ <u>Your Treatment is:</u>

❑ Physical Therapy   *(see chapter 5)*

❑ MRI

❑ X-ray

❑ Injection of Kenalog   *(see chapter 7)*

❑ Arthroscopic Surgery: *(see chapter 4)*

      ○ Repair of tendon tear

      ○ Cleaning of bursa

      ○ Smoothing of bone spur

      ○ Smoothing of AC Joint

      ○ Repair SLAP

      ○ Cleaning SLAP

      ○ Repair of Labrum

      ○ Release of scarred lining

❑ MUA (manipulation under anesthesia)

❑ Other: _____

☤ *Web RX for Patient Education:*

Web site: *www.RoacheMD.com*

Choose: Patient Education

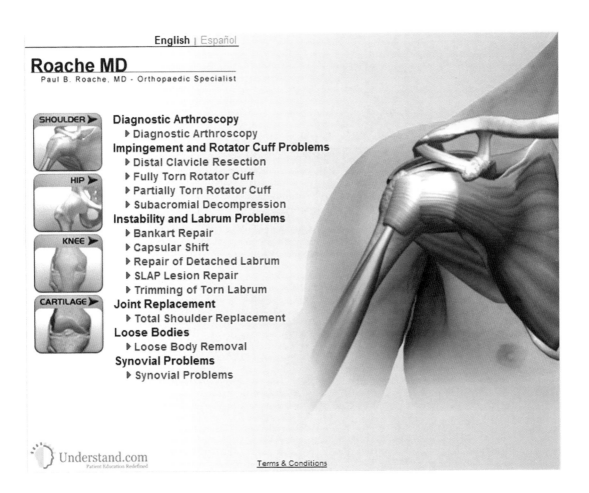

Table of Contents

Other Approaches

Appendices

Why I Wrote This Handbook and Why You Should Read It

This handbook is the result of the countless conversations I've had with my patients about their rotator cuff injuries and other common shoulder problems. Their desire to understand their injury and the how to heal from that injury is the inspiration for this handbook.

I've written it in everyday language to convey basic terms and concepts. As such, it is a simplification; yet it is from these basic, simple concepts that injuries are best understood.

Understanding the basics of your injury, the treatment, and the process of healing, will help you to ease your anxiety and focus your energy on getting well. This book is the bridge to the basic concepts and treatment principles that you must learn and understand in order to have a meaningful conversation with your doctor.

There are many ways to treat shoulder pain and injuries. There are numerous books for patients published on the rotator cuff by chiropractors, physical therapists, and yoga teachers. Yet there are none published by shoulder surgeons for their patients.

My goal for each and every patient is that he or she heals and gets back to all the activities in his or her life in the safest, most efficient way. Many times that is not surgery. However, in rotator cuff problems, particularly tendon tears, surgery at some point is very often the correct tool to help patients return to their previous level of activity. Most patients will follow a very predictable path as they heal from their injury. I call it the "Rotator Cuff Pathway." When patients understand the basics of their injury and the treatment, there is much less fear and anxiety. Most find the predictability of the pathway reassuring. Then they are free to focus their energy on healing and getting well.

I hope this book helps you with understanding your injury and speeds you to recovery.

Paul B. Roache, MD

CHAPTER 1:

Basic Anatomy and Function of the Shoulder

◈ Key Questions

- ❏ What is the rotator cuff?
- ❏ What is a tendon?

What is the rotator cuff?

In general, when we are talking about the rotator cuff we are talking about the four essential muscles, and their tendons, of the shoulder. These are the most important elements of the shoulder socket and are critical for a healthy, well functioning shoulder.

What is a tendon?

A tendon is strong tissue that connects muscles to bone. When muscles contract, they pull on tendon and thereby pull on the bone. Tendon is the body's version of rope. Because of the tendon, when muscles contract, we are able to move.

◈ Key Concept

The shoulder is a ball-and-socket joint but with a special socket.

Three things make the shoulder socket special:

1. The socket is mostly made of the rotator cuff. Most of the soft tissues of the socket are the muscle and tendon of the rotator cuff. The rest are the ligaments and joint lining of the socket, called the capsule.

2. <u>The socket has a hard roof.</u> The bone and ligament of the arch over the rotator cuff provide support for the tendons as they slide in the socket. There is an important pad to cushion the tendons from the hard roof called a **bursa**.

3. <u>The socket is mobile.</u> The scapula (shoulder blade) is the bony foundation of the socket. The scapula and the socket it supports are mobile. This gives the shoulder a tremendous range of motion. This motion requires coordination and balance of the muscles around the shoulder, particularly the rotator cuff.

Details

<u>The socket is mostly made of the rotator cuff.</u>

Four muscles and their tendons make up the rotator cuff. The tendons of the rotator cuff muscles are woven together and truly create a **cuff** of tendon around the ball (proximal humerus) by their attachments to the ball (greater and lesser tuberosities). This is much like the cuff of a shirtsleeve. This cuff of tendons is essential for **rotation** of the ball. This is why they are called the "**rotator**" **cuff.** These **rotator cuff tendons** are the key part of the socket.

These tendons surround the ball on three sides. Essentially, it is a three-sided box with one muscle on the front, one on the top, and two on the back. There are no rotator cuff muscles on the floor. (See figure 1-1.)

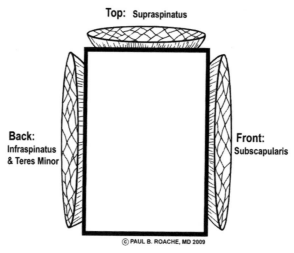

Figure 1-1a: The rotator cuff forms the three sides of a box.

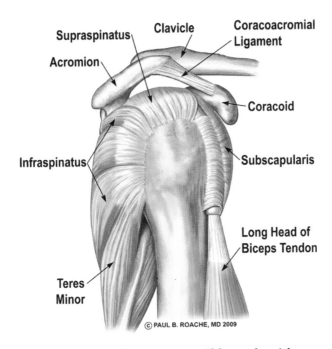

Figure 1-1b: The rotator cuff from the side.

In the front is the subscapularis muscle and tendon. On the top is the supraspinatus muscle and tendon. (See figure 1-2.)

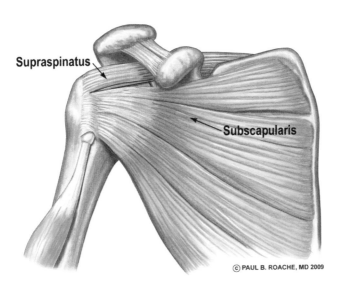

Figure 1-2: The front and top of the rotator cuff

In the back are the infrapsinatus and teres minor muscles and their tendons. (See figure 1-3.)

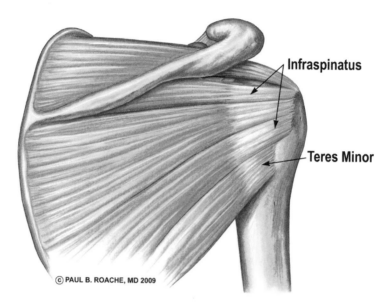

Figure 1-3: The back of the rotator cuff

The socket has a hard roof.

The hard arched roof over the tendon and bursa is made of a ligament between two bony parts of the shoulder blade.

This ligament creates an outlet for the tendons of the rotator cuff to move in and out of the space created by the hard roof. (The ligament is the coracoacromial ligament from the coracoid tip to the under surface of the acromion and AC joint). (See figure 1-4.)

You must understand a couple of key concepts about this outlet:

First, there is contact between the rotator cuff and the arch as the tendons move in and out of the outlet. *This contact is normal.* The rotator cuff and its bursa slide under this arch as the muscles of the rotator cuff contract and shorten or lengthen.

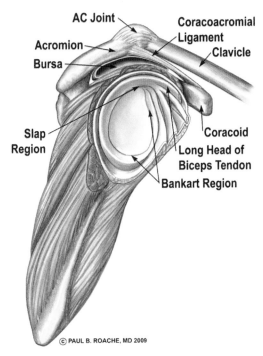

Figure 1-4: The outlet for the rotator cuff and its hard roof

Second, the arch is hard. As tissues move in and out of this outlet, they slide across the hard edge of the arch. This hard edge is cushioned by the bursa, which is the body's version of a pad (subacromial bursa in this case). (See figure 1-5a.)

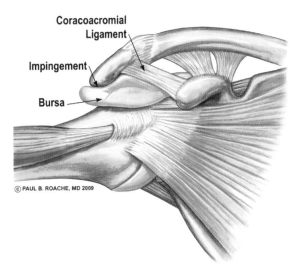

Figure 1-5a: Subacromial bursa cushioning the rotator cuff

The hard edge can pinch or catch the bursa and the rotator cuff. This is abnormal contact and is called outlet impingement. Abnormal contact can cause the bursa to become inflamed (irritated). This can be very painful. If it persists over a period of time, the arch will develop a thicker ligament and bursa. This is similar to developing a callus on your hand from repeated contact. Sometimes bone will form in the ligament as a response to this forceful contact. This is called a **bone spur** (See Figure 1-5b.)

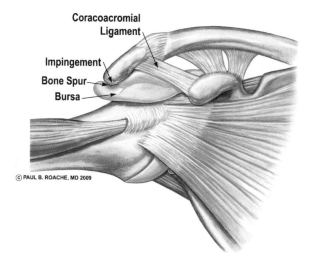

Figure 1-5b: Bone spur in the subacromial space causing impingement

When impingement at the outlet persists, the rotator cuff can tear in response to this abnormal contact. (See Figure 1-5c.)

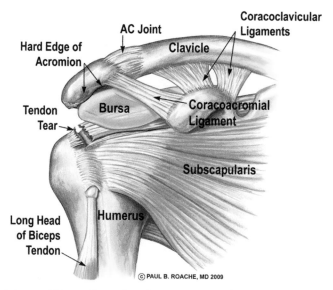

Figure 1-5c: A rotator cuff tear, from impingement at the outlet and the key anatomy.

<u>The socket is mobile.</u>

The shoulder has amazing range of motion—more than any other joint in the body. This is because the socket on the shoulder blade (scapula) is able to rotate, tilt, and move forward, backward, up, and down. (See Figure 1-6.)

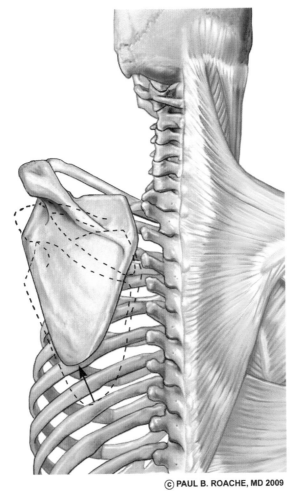

© PAUL B. ROACHE, MD 2009

Figure 1-6: Movement of the shoulder blade (scapula) when you "shrug" your shoulder

The coordination of the muscles of the rotator cuff and the other shoulder muscles makes this possible. This mobility is also why the shoulder is vulnerable to injury. All these moving parts, in essence, can break down. When they do, it can dramatically affect the way the shoulder functions.

Let's briefly look at the key parts of the shoulder.

◇ **Key Anatomy**

Basics: (things you need to know)

■ **Bones**

Three bones make up the shoulder: (See figures 1-5c and 1-6)
- ❏ Clavicle (**collarbone**)
- ❏ Scapula (**shoulder blade**—socket lives here)
- ❏ Humerus (**ball of the socket**)

■ **Joints**

These bones create **three joints and one pseudo joint** (by definition a joint is the meeting point of two bones): (See Figure 1-7)

- ❏ The sternoclavicular joint (**SC joint**) – This connects the clavicle (collarbone) to the sternum (breast bone).
- ❏ The acromioclavicular joint (**AC joint**) – This connects the clavicle (collarbone) to the scapula (shoulder blade) at the superior portion called the acromion.
- ❏ The glenohumeral joint (**GH joint**) – This connects the humerus (ball) to the scapula at the lateral portion called the glenoid (socket). This is the main joint of the shoulder and the ball and socket discussed above.

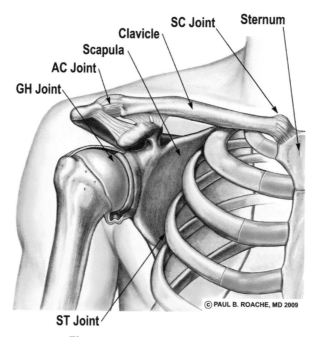

Figure 1-7: Joints of the Shoulder

❑ The scapulothoracic joint (**ST joint**) – The scapula, the muscle of the sub-scapularis, the posterior ribs, and intercostal muscles of the posterior thorax move over each other in a joint-like fashion, but it is not a true joint.

• • •

Extra Credit: (for those who want more)

Details

The clavicle (collarbone) is an S-shaped, tubular bone that is approximately six to eight inches in length. It is the only bony connection of the shoulder and the arm to the skeleton. It has three main movements: elevation, depression (up and down like a lever arm), and rotation. The majority of this movement occurs at the SC joint. The SC joint has two sets of very strong ligaments that keep the joint stable and allow it to perform its normal motion. (These are called costoclavicular ligaments).

The clavicle acts not only as a lever arm for the shoulder, but also as a protective shield to the important nerves that run from the neck to the arm. The clavicle is the only bony connection of the spine and thorax to the arm. This occurs at the AC joint. This joint is held in place by two sets of ligaments to the outside end of the clavicle (the coracoclavicular ligaments and AC ligaments). This is important to know when discussing injuries to the clavicle and the AC joint (See also Chapter 12).

Finally, the scapula moves on the posterior chest wall. The ST joint, although this is not a typical joint, has some characteristics of a joint and, thus, can have some of the problems that a joint may have (bursitis, and so forth).

■ Muscles

Seventeen muscles comprise the shoulder. These muscles are divided into three groups. (See Figures 1-8a and 1-8b)

Scapula to humerus: nine muscles
  ❑ The **rotator cuff has four muscles.** (See Figures 1-2 and 1-3.)
  ❑ The deltoid muscle has three parts, but it is one muscle.
  ❑ There are four non-rotator cuff muscles: teres major, triceps, biceps, and coracobracialis.

Skeleton to scapula: six muscles
- ❑ Pectoralis minor
- ❑ Trapezious
- ❑ Levator scapula
- ❑ Serratus
- ❑ Rhomboid major
- ❑ Rhomboid minor

Skeleton to humerus: two muscles
- ❑ Pectoralis major
- ❑ Latissimus dorsi (Occasionally, part of the latissimus attaches to the scapula in some patients.)

LATISSIMUS DORSI & TRAPEZIUS

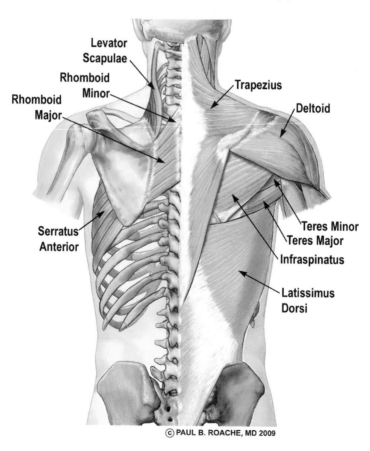

© PAUL B. ROACHE, MD 2009

Figure 1-8a: The muscles of the shoulder from the back

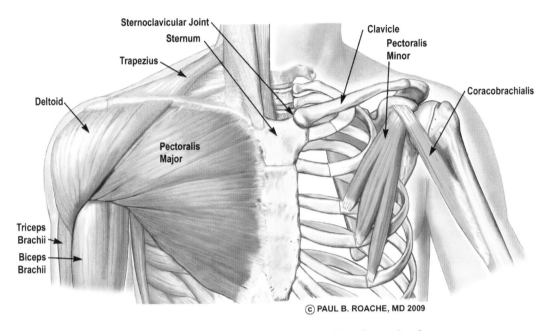

Figure 1-8b: The muscles of the shoulder from the front

■ Nerves

In simple terms, nerves are the body's version of wire, and carry the electrical signals from the brain that direct the muscles to perform their actions. They also carry the signals of pain, and send signals of position to the brain. (See Figure 1-9) In the shoulder, six nerve roots come from the neck. Five of these combine into a nerve center for the shoulder and arm called the brachial plexus. The brachial plexus then gives off multiple nerves that operate the muscles of the shoulder and give sensation to the region.

The two most important nerves to the shoulder are the suprascapular nerve and the axillary nerve.

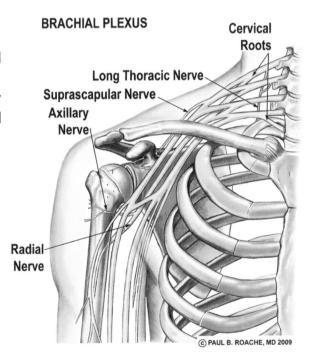

Figure 1-9: The key nerves of the shoulder from the neck and brachial plexus

◇ Key Function

The main role of the shoulder is to position the hand. This is why shoulder problems often present as problems of activity. For example, difficulties with combing your hair, brushing your teeth, eating, getting dressed, working with your hands overhead, throwing a ball, and so forth.

The key muscles of the shoulder for elevating the arm are the rotator cuff muscles.

The rotator cuff functions as a unit.

As a unit, the rotator cuff has only one main function: **keep the ball centered in the socket.** This is very important to give the arm a pivot point for elevating and/or rotating the arm. If you think of the ball and socket as similar to a golf ball on a tee, but surrounded by the rotator cuff, you will understand the basic function of the rotator cuff. No matter how the ball rotates, the muscles pull and keep tension on the ball. (See Fig 1-10)

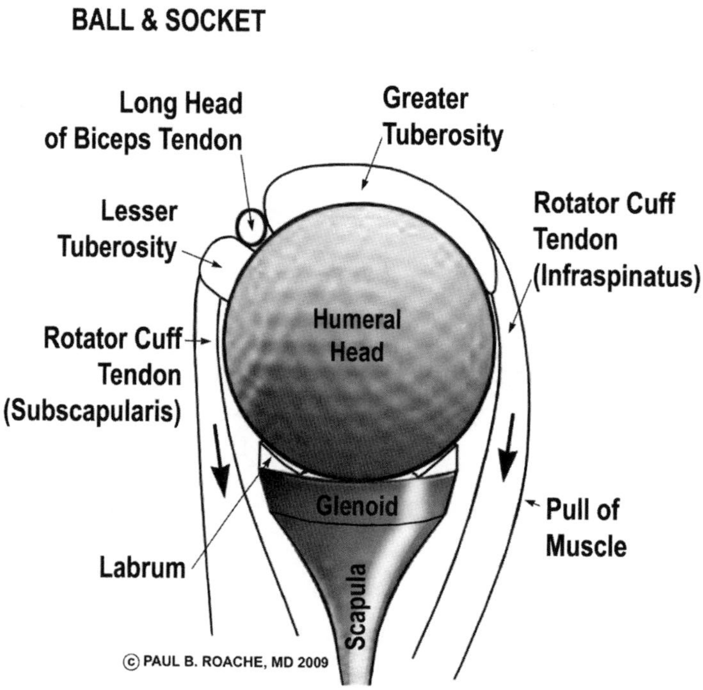

BALL & SOCKET

Long Head of Biceps Tendon — Greater Tuberosity — Lesser Tuberosity — Rotator Cuff Tendon (Infraspinatus) — Rotator Cuff Tendon (Subscapularis) — Humeral Head — Glenoid — Pull of Muscle — Labrum — Scapula

© PAUL B. ROACHE, MD 2009

Fig: 1-10: The ball and socket (aka golf ball on tee)

The rotator cuff has two secondary functions: **assist in rotation and elevation of the arm** at the shoulder joint.

These functions allow us to perform most of our activities of daily life, for example reaching for door knobs, reaching for jars on the top of a shelf, and so forth.

All other muscles of the shoulder girdle are important for positioning the scapula and arm during activities.

• • •

◈ Summary

There are four key points to remember about the shoulder and rotator cuff.

1. It is a ball-and-socket joint, but the socket is mostly soft tissue.
2. The socket is mobile and requires balance and muscle coordination.
3. The rotator cuff's main function is to center the ball and keep it rolling.
4. The rotator cuff's secondary function is to assist in rotation and elevation.

If you understand these four keys, then understanding the spectrum of injuries to the rotator cuff and shoulder girdle becomes manageable.

Now let's look at common shoulder injuries.

CHAPTER 2

Rotator Cuff Injury and Treatment Basics

◇ Key Questions

- ❑ How is the rotator cuff injured?
- ❑ How do you know there is an injury?
- ❑ Does a rotator cuff tear heal?
- ❑ What can be done to treat the injury?

Basics: (things you need to know)

How is the rotator cuff injured?

The majority of injuries to the rotator cuff are "wear and tear" type of injuries to the soft tissue of the socket. Most patients cannot remember a specific event where the pain and problem began. Most commonly, the pain is at a low level at first and barely gets in the way of normal activities. Patients seek help when the pain gets in the way of sleep, sports, or daily activities.

How do you know there is an injury?

◇ Common Symptoms

Pain:

Shoulder pain is the most common symptom in rotator cuff injuries. ***Pain that interrupts sleep is also very common.*** Pain can range from a dull ache at rest to a sharp pain with activities that elevate the arm. It can radiate to the neck, the front, the back, and the side of the shoulder. It often radiates down the outside of the arm as well. Although we don't yet fully understand the pain mechanisms in the shoulder, the bursa appears to be a major source of pain signals.

Pinching and pain with elevation of the arm:
Pain and pinching or catching when you elevate your arm above the shoulder can be signs of impingement. (See chapter 1, figure 1-5b)
This can vary from a low level ache to a forceful sharp pain.

Weakness and motion loss:
Weakness while elevating the arm is the second most common symptom reported. Some patients with very large tears cannot elevate their arm at all. Loss of ability to elevate the arm can also be related to stiffness in the shoulder, sometimes known as frozen shoulder.

Evaluation by Shoulder Specialist:
The correct diagnosis is essential for deciding upon proper treatment. This requires a surgeon who is experienced in the history, examination, and imaging of the shoulder.

When the history and examination indicate that there is a rotator cuff injury, it is often time for imaging of the shoulder. X-rays, MRI, and ultrasound are commonly used to evaluate the rotator cuff.

X-rays are usually required to help make the diagnosis. (See Figure 2-1.) X-rays show bony structures very well, but do not show tendon. Often these X-rays are normal, but they can provide a wealth of information about the overall structure and health of the joint.

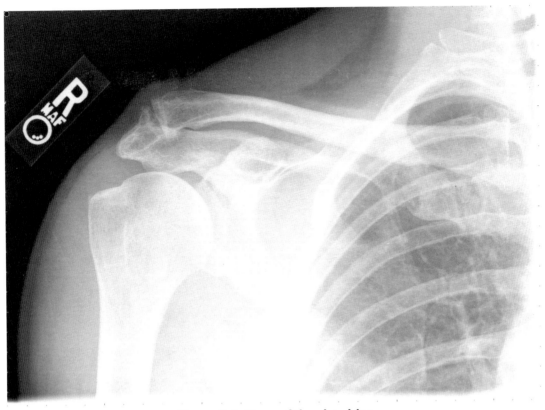

Figure 2-1: X-ray of the shoulder

MRI (magnetic resonance imaging) is frequently used to gain more information about the shoulder. (See Figure 2-2.) It is a more advanced method for imaging all the structures in the shoulder. It is especially good at showing the tendons, muscles, and ligaments.

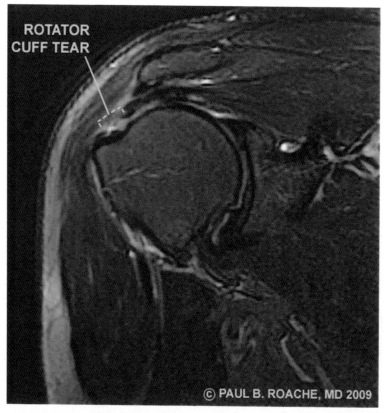

Figure 2-2: MRI of shoulder demonstrating a tear in the rotator cuff)

Ultrasound is increasingly being used in the office to evaluate rotator cuff injuries and their healing after surgery. However, its accuracy and, therefore, its usefulness are dependent on the experience and skill of the surgeon.

Does a rotator cuff tendon tear heal?

The current published literature has some important data that guides the surgeon in making an early surgical decision to treat rotator cuff injuries.

- ❑ Inflammation can heal
- ❑ Chronic tears do not seem to heal on their own.
- ❑ Existing tears have a 50 percent chance of becoming larger.
- ❑ Full tendon tears are directly related to progression of muscle atrophy and fatty infiltration. This can lead to permanent weakness and dysfunction.

While there may be a few acute tears that can heal on their own, the overwhelming majority of tears will not heal. In fact, many will get bigger over the one to two years after the diagnosis is first made.

Why don't torn tendons of the rotator cuff heal?

The biggest reason seems to be that the blood supply is interrupted when the tendon is pulled away from its bony attachment. This is also why more than 50 percent of these tears will become larger over two years. While this may sound discouraging, there are a couple of things to consider. First, even though a torn tendon may not heal, the rotator cuff works as a unit, and the remaining tendons can compensate for the torn part of the tendon. This is often achieved with the help of a physical therapist. Second, even though 50 percent of tears will become larger, the rotator cuff can compensate, so even enlarging tears have shown the ability to maintain good function.

However, when full shoulder function is not restored and there is continued pain, it is time to consider a surgical repair.

What can be done to treat the injury?

◇ Treatment Basics

<u>Treat Inflammation and rebalance shoulder:</u>

- ❑ Oral medication: nonsteroidal anti-inflammatory (ibuprofen, etc.)
- ❑ Subacromial bursa injection with a steroid anti-inflammatory (1 to 2cc of Kenalog, etc.) to heal inflammation, if there is significant pain and/or a positive impingement sign.
- ❑ Four to six weeks of physical therapy for rotator cuff training
- ❑ If there is no significant improvement, consider surgical treatment.

<u>Oral Medicines</u>

The most commonly used oral medicines are the non-steroidal anti-inflammatory class of medications. These medicines include Motrin (Ibuprofen), Naprosyn, and so forth. These medicines are very good at reducing low-level inflammation. Consult your medical doctor if you have high blood pressure or a history of stomach ulcers before you use these medications.

<u>Physical Therapy</u>

The overall goals of physical therapy are to:

1. Increase strength and coordination of the rotator cuff and supporting scapular muscles

2. Increase motion
3. Decrease pain and inflammation.

The physical therapist has many tools to achieve these goals. (See Chapter 5.)

Injections

Steroid anti-inflammatory medications like Cortisone or Kenalog can be injected directly into the bursa. This is a very powerful and effective treatment for healing moderate to severe inflammation. Research has shown these injections to be very safe and have very few side effects. The positive results in many patients can be nothing short of dramatic. (See Chapter 7 for common myths about injections.)

Surgical Treatments

When surgery is needed, it is directed toward two primary goals. First, eliminate the mechanical causes of pain and inflammation (for example, bone spurs). Second, stimulate a healing response in the repaired tendon. (See later in this chapter.)

◇ Key concept

<u>Understanding the Injury</u>

Injuries to the rotator cuff and shoulder occur in two categories:
- ❑ Direct
- ❑ Indirect

There are <u>four main</u> groups of <u>direct injuries</u> to the rotator cuff:

1. Inflammatory injuries of the bursa and tendon
2. Impingement injuries (pinching of the bursa and tendon)
3. Abrasion or partial tearing of the tendon
4. Complete tearing of the tendon

Let's look at the four main groups of direct injuries.

<u>Inflammation</u>

The bursa in the socket is a pad. Contact in the socket is normal. However, if contact is too heavy, the bursa will produce fluid to add cushioning and padding at contact points. When the bursa becomes inflamed, the inflammation can have momentum of its own. It can continue even after the initial cause has resolved. Inflammation is part of the body's normal healing response, but it can continue longer than needed and be quite painful.

The tendons can also become inflamed. Usually this occurs in conjunction with in-flammation of the bursa. When the tendon is inflamed, it can swell but otherwise be intact. The lining of the socket can become inflamed as well (see Chapter 6: Frozen Shoulder).

<u>Impingement (Outlet Impingement)</u>

Contact in the ball and socket is a normal occurrence. (See Figure 2-3.) However, there are points around the edge where there is a transition from soft to hard structures, and these points can pinch the cuff or bursa. When that occurs, pain and inflammation can start. If the pinching goes on long enough or with enough force, it can cause abrasion or even tearing of the rotator cuff.

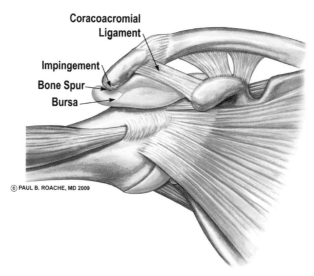

Figure 2-3: Impingement of the rotator cuff

Abrasion and Partial Tearing

When pinching of the tendon has been present long enough, injury will start to occur. This is similar to a door rubbing on carpet and wearing it down. The tendon injury can be from direct rubbing or from tension when the cuff is pinched. Direct contact can injure the tendon on the bursal side of the tendon. It can also stop the normal movement of the tendon on the superficial layers and result in increased tension on the deep side of the tendon. (See Figure 2-4.)

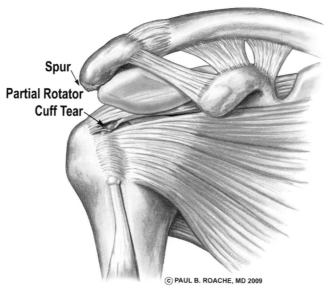

Figure 2-4: Partial tendon tear of the rotator cuff.

Complete Tears

When the tendon is detached from the ball, we call this a complete tear. (See Figure 2-5.) They come in a range of sizes and configuration.

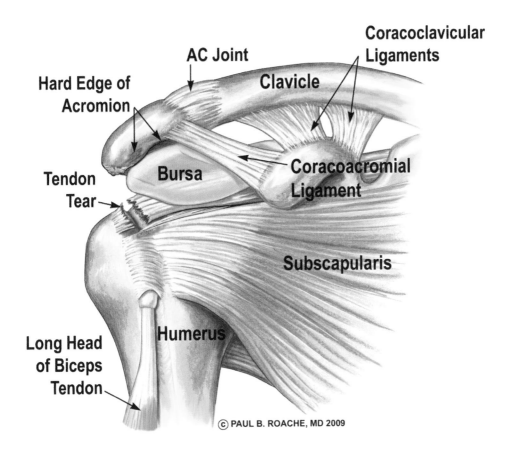

Figure 2-5: Complete tendon tear of the rotator cuff.

• • •

Extra Credit: (for those who want more)

In addition, there are <u>three secondary</u> groups of injuries that affect the rotator cuff <u>indirectly</u>.

1. Pain inhibition
2. Neurological dysfunction
3. Systemic disorders

Pain inhibition:
Pain generated from an injury of the shoulder can send signals to the muscles of the shoulder to limit activity. During an examination, this can test like a rotator cuff tear. When the injury heals or is treated the muscle no longer receives the signal of an injury and returns to full activity. This is common with impingement and bursal inflammation. It is also common after surgery.

Neurological dysfunction:

Nerve dysfunction is perhaps the most complicated problem in shoulder injuries. The nerves around the shoulder and those that come from the neck can be involved with a shoulder injury. Sometimes they are simply irritated and inflamed. Sometimes they have been pinched by the muscle spasm. Occasionally, they have been stretched or torn.

It can be a challenge to determine whether shoulder injury is the cause of neck and nerve pain; or neck and nerve injury are the cause of shoulder pain. Large rotator cuff tears are associated with nerve injury to the suprascapular nerve. This can affect the recovery after surgery. Nerve injuries to the suprascapular nerve can mimic a large rotator cuff tear. (see chapter 10)

Systemic Disorders:
Diseases of the soft tissue such as Rheumatoid Arthritis can predispose the rotator cuff to tear and complicate surgical repair. Diabetes can predispose a patient for sustained inflammation. The microvascular disease associated with diabetes can weaken the tendons of the rotator cuff.

These three secondary injuries require the expertise of your doctor to assess and treat.

CHAPTER 3:

Understanding Surgical Treatment of Rotator Cuff Injuries

<u>The three keys</u> to remember are:

1. Torn tendons do not heal back to the bone on their own.
2. 50 percent of tears will become larger in two years.
3. Surgical Treatment is 85 to 90 percent successful at restoring function.

Basics: (things you need to know)

◇ Surgical Treatments

When conservative therapies have not helped heal a patient with a rotator cuff injury, surgery is usually needed to restore normal function. Surgery is simply a therapeutic tool to help patients heal. It is directed toward two primary goals. <u>First</u>, eliminate the mechanical causes of pain and inflammation (for example, bone spurs). <u>Second</u>, repair the tendon to bone and stimulate a healing response.

In order to achieve these goals, surgeons have many excellent tools to use. The arthroscope is one of my main tools. It allows me to enter the shoulder joint through very small, quarter inch incisions and navigate the space with very little irritation to the normal tissues. Essentially, it is a video camera with a long, tubular lens. The arthroscope provides a detailed view of the shoulder anatomy. With the arthroscope, bone spurs are easy to treat and tendon tears are readily seen and treated. (See Figure 3-1.) On my Web site's patient education section, there are excellent pictures to help patients understand the basics of the arthroscopic surgery for a rotator cuff tear. (See Patient Education Web RX: Fully Torn Rotator Cuff.)

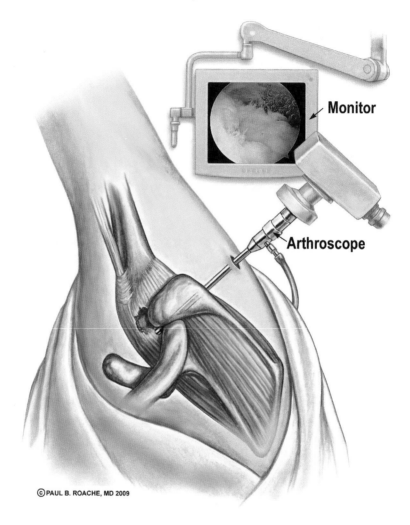

© PAUL B. ROACHE, MD 2009

Figure 3-1: The arthroscope in the shoulder

Surgical treatments are grouped into four main categories:
A. Decompression of the subacromial space
B. Repair of torn tendon(s) in the rotator cuff
C. Biceps tendon treatment: repair, release, and reattachment
D. AC Joint Resection

Decompression of the Subacromial Space

This includes removal of bone spurs and cleaning out tissue that is getting pinched. Essentially, this procedure makes more room for the tendon and smoothes the edges so there is no longer pinching. (See Figures 3-2a, 3-2b, 3-3a and 3-3b)

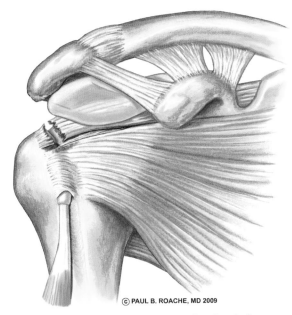

Figure 3-2a: The drawing of Bone Spur in the Subacromial Space

ACROMIOPLASTY

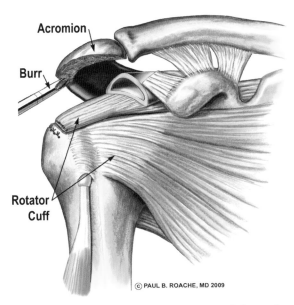

Figure 3-2b: The drawing of the Decompression of the Subacromial Space

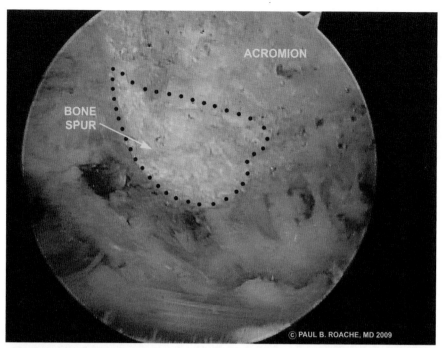

Figure 3-3a: The view from the arthroscope of the bone spur in the Subacromial Space

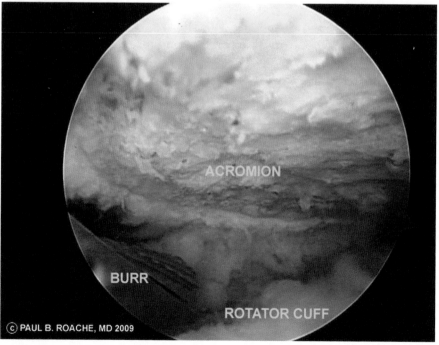

Figure 3-3b: The view from the arthroscope after the Decompression of the Subacromial Space. (Smoothing the edges and bone spurs) Note the space created.

• • •

Repair of Torn Tendon(s) in the Rotator Cuff.

When the tendon needs to be "repaired," this essentially means that it needs to be sewn to bone. The stitches will hold it while it heals back to bone. (See Figures 3-4a, 3-4b, 3-5a, and 3-5b)

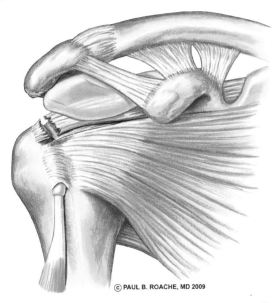

Figure 3-4a: The drawing of the torn rotator cuff tendon

REPAIR OF
ROTATOR CUFF

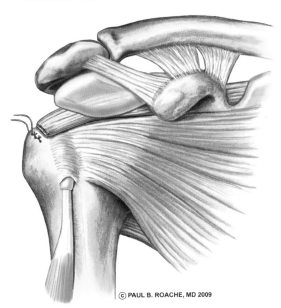

Figure 3-4b: The drawing of the repaired rotator cuff tendon

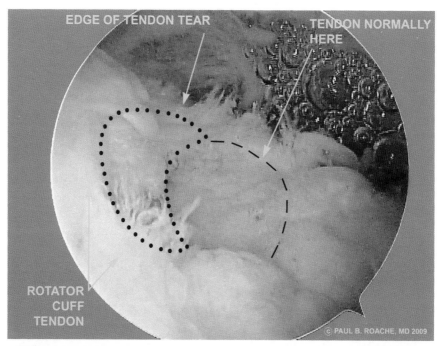

Figure 3-5a:The arthroscopic view of the torn rotator cuff tendon

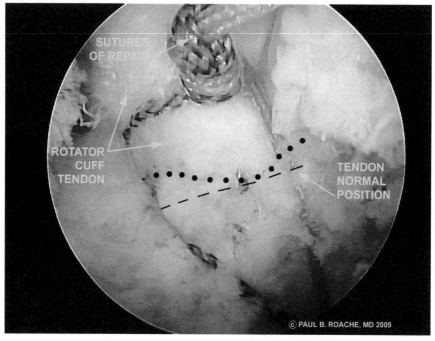

Figure 3-5b: The arthroscopic view of repaired rotator cuff tendon

• • •

The technical details of a rotator cuff repair are the source of endless discussions at many meetings I attend. Primarily, there are three available techniques.

1. Arthroscopic assisted repair
2. Mini-open repair
3. Traditional open repair

No matter which technique is selected, the biology of healing remains the same. All three techniques have very good long term results. The arthroscopic technique has the advantage of less discomfort for patients in the period immediately after surgery.

The goal is the same no matter which technique is chosen. As the surgeon I should achieve a solid repair of the tendon back to bone and stimulate a healing response.

In my opinion, ten elements affect the quality of repairs and the ultimate result.

1. The size of the tear—smaller tears simply do better
2. The quality and mobility of the tendon
3. The quality of the bone to which the tendon will be reattached
4. The blood supply to the area of repair (The health of the patient is very important to the quality of the blood supply. Cardiovascular fitness is a big help for healing. Smoking is absolutely a problem for healing.)
5. Achieving a repair that recreates the anatomy and normal tension of the tendon attachment
6. The number of stitch strands crossing the repair and the configuration and strength of the stitches
7. Strict use of an external-rotation sling in the first six weeks to protect the repair and the healing tissue
8. A *Protected Early Motion Program* (Phase 1) to prevent stiffness and lubricate the joint. This phase of rehabilitation starts before surgery, with the teaching of the important exercises, which will need to start after surgery. This is called pre-habilitation or "Prehab". (See chapter 5)
9. An experienced physical therapist to oversee the three phases of rehabilitation
10. Delaying strengthening exercises for eight to twelve weeks in order to protect the repair and the healing tissue

In addition to keeping yourself as healthy as possible, I think keeping positive mental and emotional outlook help speed the recovery.

Surgical Results

In general terms, rotator cuff surgery is extremely successful. Long-term studies on traditional open rotator cuff repairs demonstrate that up to 90 percent of patients report significant functional improvement and lessening of pain at greater than seven years after surgery. Mini-open and arthroscopic-assisted repairs have shown very similar results in recent studies.

I typically choose the arthroscopic approach in small- and medium-size tears and some very large tears. The main advantages of arthroscopic repairs are decreased potential injury to the deltoid and decreased pain in the immediate period after the repair. What most patients notice is that there are four or five very small (half-inch) incision scars instead of a single four-inch scar for the open approach.

Biceps Tendon Surgical Treatments:

The Biceps tendon can be a source of pain and dysfunction for many patients. This can be the result of chronic injury from the tendon rubbing on the biceps groove. It can also be from traumatic injury. If the tendon or its attachment into the SLAP region is injured significantly, then treatment is needed. (See Chapter 9: SLAP Tears and Biceps Tendon Injuries.)
Surgeons have known for some time that simply releasing the tendon can relieve the pain. We can live and function normally without a Biceps tendon; however, some patients will notice a balling up of the biceps called "Popeye deformity." Even though it will cause no functional problem, most patients prefer not to have a "Popeye deformity." Therefore, in most cases, I reattach the biceps tendon to a location that will not cause pain after it has healed. As a note, periodically we hear about athletes (usually quarterbacks) who tear their biceps and feel better.

AC Joint Resection/Surgical Treatments:

Some patients will have significant pain at the distal end of the clavicle. A simple trimming of the distal end of the bone to prevent it from rubbing and causing pain is a very effective way to treat this source of pain. I usually do it at the same time that I am performing the subacromial decompression. (See Figure 3-6)

MUMFORD

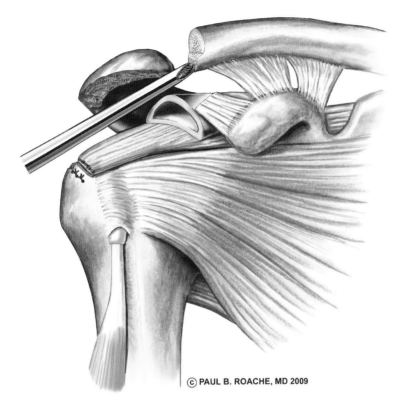

© PAUL B. ROACHE, MD 2009

Figure 3-6: Distal Clavicle resection or Mumford

• • •

Extra Credit: (for those who want more)

<u>Special Problems</u>

Just a few words on these two uncommon problems:

A. Tears that are not repairable
B. Tears that lead to arthritis

These problems are not common. In general, there are four treatment paths.

1. Pain relief with injections or arthroscopic debridement (cleaning of the space above the tear) and biceps tenotomy (releasing the biceps tendon)
2. Pain relief from a hemiarthroplasty (partial joint replacement) (See Chapter 14)

3. Pain relief and partial function recovery with tendon transfers (moving the latissimus tendon)

4. Pain relief and partial function recovery with the reverse ball-and-socket prosthesis (a newly FDA-approved joint-replacement device, which can be very effective for certain patients)(See Chapter 14)

Note: The reverse ball-and-socket prosthesis has been used successfully for many years in Europe. My first experience with it was in 1999 while visiting Zurich. It has been in use in the United States for several years. It provides certain patients with a treatment that can have dramatic benefits, but it also has approximately a 20 percent complication rate. You should consult your shoulder surgeon for further information.

CHAPTER 4:

Getting Ready for Shoulder Surgery, An Overview

Once you have decided to have surgery, the organized preparation for the surgery begins. If you become familiar with the process, it will help you relieve any anxiety that can naturally come with having surgery. Equally important is to understand the steps of the pathway to full healing after surgery. If you know where you are going, it will help you relax and focus on your recovery.

◇ **Keys Questions:**

- ❑ **How will your surgery be scheduled?**
- ❑ **What is your injury and what is the surgical plan to treat your injury?**
- ❑ **What are the risks and benefits of the surgery?**
- ❑ **What should you know about anesthesia?**
- ❑ **How should you prepare for surgery?**
- ❑ **What can you expect immediately after surgery?**
- ❑ **How do you recognize problems immediately after surgery?**
- ❑ **How long will it take to heal and get well?**
- ❑ **A note on discomfort after surgery.**

How will your surgery be scheduled?
The Surgery Scheduler will coordinate everything that is necessary to get ready for surgery. In general it takes 3-4 weeks to go through the process. Any questions about the process, the scheduler can answer.

In general the process is:

1. Your insurance will be contacted to authorize the surgery.
2. The surgery will be scheduled. Keep in mind that the schedule is subject to change due to emergencies or operating room schedule changes.
3. The pre-surgery checklist and information will be sent by mail (see appendix B).
4. If you have medical problems you will see your primary care doctor to get clearance. This is to ensure your safety for surgery.
5. You will meet with your Physical Therapist before surgery to plan your rehabilitation.
6. Pain medications, and possibly an ice machine, will be arranged.

What is your injury and what is the surgical plan to treat your injury?
Understanding your problem and why surgery is necessary to heal that problem is important. Know and understand your diagnosis and the surgical plan.
You can review the basic information of your injury and planned surgery in this handbook and on my website: www.RoacheMD.com. (See WebRX in the front of this handbook)

What are the risks and benefits of the surgery?
The risks of surgery are important to understand before surgery. Overall, surgery is very safe. Arthroscopic surgery is, in general, even safer and is performed as outpatient surgery. So, you will go home shortly after you wake up.

A few key facts to understand about arthroscopic surgery and surgery risks:
- ❑ The success rate of most arthroscopic surgeries is greater than 85 percent.
- ❑ Infections are very rare, less than one in four hundred cases. You will get antibiotics at the time of surgery, which is the best protection. If an infection occurs, further surgery is required with prolonged treatment with antibiotics.
- ❑ Swelling from the sterile fluid used for the arthroscopic surgery (particularly in the shoulder) is expected. Occasionally, observation overnight is needed while the swelling diminishes.
- ❑ Complications from arthroscopic surgery are rare. Possible complications include unexpected findings at time of surgery, failure of a device or the procedure, and injury to normal structures.
- ❑ Serious complications are very rare. Deep Venous Thrombosis (blood clots) can form during or after surgery. Although rare, a DVT is very serious. Patients with previous history are of DVT are at greater risk.

❑ Modern anesthesia is very safe for healthy patients. Some patients with medical problems will need to have their surgery at the hospital to ensure their safety.

❑ Shoulder stiffness postoperatively from shoulder arthroscopy is common. It is essential to follow the exercise program as specified to minimize this problem. If you develop stiffness, it will prolong the rehabilitation and recovery time.

What should you know about anesthesia?

Overview of Anesthesia by Bill Spina, MD

Patients will often receive a combination of anesthesia—a regional anesthesia or local anesthesia and a general anesthesia. A regional anesthesia in the shoulder called an "interscalene block." This works much like when a dentist gives a patient Novocain to numb the operative area. The anesthesiologist will inject medicine into the area above the clavicle containing the nerves going to the shoulder/arm. This injection can make the area "go to sleep" or feel numb for up to twelve to sixteen hours. A light general anesthesia is usually also given. It is usually most comfortable for you to be asleep during the surgery.

If a regional anesthesia is used, you will need less general anesthesia. Often when you wake up, you will have little or no pain. On the day of surgery you will discuss this with your anesthesiologist and see if a regional anesthesia is appropriate for you.

How should you prepare for surgery?

Optimizing your health before surgery is very important. The better your health before surgery, the better the healing process will proceed. This may seem obvious, but for most patients, it is not always easy to change health habits. In essence, consider yourself in training for healing after surgery.

Key steps to take before your surgery:
❑ Adopt a positive mental attitude! Reduce stress. Your body knows how to heal.
❑ Keeping your muscles in shape and your joints flexible will speed recovery.
❑ Cardiovascular exercise and fitness improve circulation and healing.
❑ **Stop Smoking**! If you can't stop, cut back. Do whatever you can, nicotine patches, etc. This alone will improve your circulation and healing.
❑ Improve your diet.

❑ Get adequate sleep and rest.
❑ Meet with your physical therapist to plan your rehabilitation.
❑ Complete the pre-surgery checklist (see appendix B)

What can you expect immediately after surgery?
(See appendix B for the detailed post-surgery checklist)

❑ You will be groggy after surgery from anesthesia. Plan to be at home for the first 24-48 hours.
❑ There will be difficulties performing basic life tasks: eating, going to the bathroom, etc. This is normal.
❑ You should shower by 48 hours after surgery and change the dressing if needed.
❑ The nurses and my office will be calling to check on you.

How do you recognize problems immediately after surgery?

❑ If pain or swelling (or both) continue or get worse, or the pain is unrelieved by the pain medication.
❑ If you notice redness or swelling, or if pus drains from the incision site.
❑ If you have a fever higher than 101.5 F in the first 7 days after surgery.
❑ If the incision site bleeds excessively.
❑ If you have a sudden onset of shortness of breath or chest pain.
❑ If you have unusual swelling and pain of you legs.

You should call my office if you have any questions or concerns.

How long will it take to heal and get well?

Know how long your recovery will take and when it is safe to start modified activities and work. Be Realistic! You can't speed it up, but you can slow it down. Complete each phase of the recovery. The body needs time to complete the healing. Stick to the program.

In general, the recovery from *shoulder arthroscopy for a rotator cuff repair is* **Four to Six Months.** There are Five Phases of recovery you must complete.

Phase 1 (zero to six weeks): Protected Motion Phase
- ❑ **Sling for comfort and protection at all times**
- ❑ Pendulum activities and scapular exercise only.
- ❑ Modified activities begin: keyboarding and working with your hands are allowed.
- ❑ Discomfort usually requires ice and pain meds, and will diminish as you approach 3-5 weeks. Sleep can be challenging.

Phase 2 (Six to twelve weeks): Motion Recovery Phase
- ❑ No Sling required.
- ❑ Physical therapy to recover normal motion of the shoulder
- ❑ Modified activities continue: Light activities of deskwork, with no lifting over 2 lbs or reaching above shoulders, can begin.
- ❑ Discomfort from therapy can require ice and pain meds. Sleep is usually improving.

Phase 3 (Twelve to eighteen weeks): Strength Recovery Phase
- ❑ Full physical therapy for strength recovery and muscle coordination
- ❑ Modified activities increase: Heavier activities are allowed, including lifting of up to 25 lbs, as well as reaching above shoulders.
- ❑ Discomfort has dropped substantially and sleep is usually normal.

Phase 4 (Eighteen to twenty-four weeks): Activity Recovery Phase
- ❑ Full Therapy or Home Therapy continues
- ❑ Progressing to all activities as tolerated except contact sports and heavy labor.
- ❑ Discomfort occasionally.

Phase 5 (More than twenty-four weeks): Activity Conditioning Phase
- ❏ All activities allowed.
- ❏ Discomfort with return to full work or activities, is common for several months until the shoulder adapts to the higher level of activity.

A note on discomfort after surgery:
It is common and normal to have some shoulder pain or discomfort during the healing phases. This is part of the shoulder rebalancing and strengthening.

This discomfort diminishes with progression through each of the healing phases.

It is particularly common in phase 5 (Activity Conditioning Phase) for those in high demand sports and very physical jobs to have 3 or more months of discomfort as the shoulder is put back to the demands of sport or work. Most patients report that this discomfort disappears after 3 months. It is important to understand this so you do not worry if there is discomfort. I am monitoring my patients' recovery, and watching for problems as they progress through the 5 phases of healing.

CHAPTER 5:

Physical Therapy for Rotator Cuff Injuries and Surgery

The overview of the game plan.

◇ **Key Questions:**

- ❑ What is a physical therapist?
- ❑ What can you expect from physical therapy?
- ❑ What is the physical therapy for a rotator cuff injury?
- ❑ What are the 3 phases of formal physical therapy after surgery?

What is a physical therapist?

A physical therapist is a licensed medical practitioner specializing in the prevention and rehabilitation of injuries caused by trauma, overuse, or a disease process. These injuries are primarily musculoskeletal (sprains, strains, overuse, trauma, disease) and neurological (stroke, spinal cord injury).

What can you expect from physical therapy?

Initially, you will meet with the physical therapist for an evaluation. This entails two parts: (1) talking with the physical therapist about your current injury, occupation, activities, medical history, and so forth, and (2) undergoing a physical examination assessing, as determined necessary, posture, joint mobility, muscle flexibility and strength, nerve function (reflexes, sensation, and so forth), and other various components.

After the evaluation, the physical therapist may start your treatment that day and/ or assign you "homework" in the form of exercises to be performed on your own to help speed the recovery process. You will be expected to perform these exercises on a regular basis in addition to attending follow-up visits with the physical therapist as prescribed by your doctor.

After the initial evaluation, you will most likely see the physical therapist for follow-up treatment sessions based on your doctor's prescription, for example, two times per week for three to six weeks. The frequency and duration of visits are based solely on your individual need for physical therapy.

The actual treatment is typically broken into two parts, although this varies greatly among different physical therapists. One part of the treatment is typically "hands-on" and may be in the form of joint mobilization (physically moving the joint to regain mobility), soft-tissue mobilization (a specific type of localized massage), or manual stretching of your muscles. This part of the treatment often also utilizes various "modalities" such as heat, ice, ultrasound (the use of sound waves to provide therapeutic effects such as deep heat or to reduce inflammation), phonophoresis (the use of ultrasound waves to locally deliver medication, such as an anti-inflammatory), iontophoresis (the use of an electrical current to locally deliver medication), or electrical stimulation (the use of electric current to provide many different effects, including pain control, muscle relaxation, or muscle strengthening).

The other part of the treatment session is some type of exercise prescribed specifically for you by the physical therapist. This may include exercises for strength, balance, gait, flexibility, agility, or movements specific to your work or athletics.

It is important to understand that the "hands-on" portion of the treatment is only meant to help reduce your current symptoms, pain, tightness, and so forth. **The most important part of physical therapy is exercise**, which will ultimately allow you to not only recover from your current injury, but also allow you to maintain good health.

What is the physical therapy for a rotator cuff injury?

Non-Surgical Pathway Physical Therapy of Rotator Cuff Injuries

Usually, the joint is mobilized to recover full motion. This is almost always the first priority. This can take many weeks of stretching. Reducing inflammation is usually a significant part of the treatment. Strengthening the rotator cuff and the muscles around the shoulder is also an integral part of non-surgical treatment. Finally, coordinating and balancing the muscles is necessary for smooth functioning of the shoulder.

Patients who require surgery will often require more physical therapy.

Surgical Pathway Physical Therapy for Rotator Cuff Repairs

There are 5 phases of healing after rotator cuff surgery.
Phase 1 (zero to six weeks): Protected Motion Phase
Phase 2 (Six to twelve weeks): Motion Recovery Phase
Phase 3 (Twelve to eighteen weeks): Strength Recovery Phase
Phase 4 (Eighteen to twenty-four weeks): Activity Recovery Phase
Phase 5 (More than twenty-four weeks): Activity Conditioning Phase

But there are only 3 phases of formal physical therapy. These match the very important first 3 phases of healing. The recovery to activity and activity conditioning (phase 4 and 5) usually require home exercises but not formal physical therapy.

What are the 3 phases of formal physical therapy after surgery?

Prehab: Presurgical teaching of Phase 1 exercises by the Physical therapist. The uses of the sling, ice or the ice unit, and adaptation of activities of daily living, are also taught BEFORE surgery.

Phase I: Protected Early Motion recovery phase (six weeks). Protect the repair in a sling or brace and use gentle, passive motions. These are instituted to keep the shoulder from getting very stiff. Active muscle contraction is avoided in this period to allow the stitches to hold the tendon to the bone without the stress of active contractions that might risk gaping of the repair or the stitches pulling out.

Phase II: Motion Recovery phase (six weeks). Here, passive stretching is accelerated to mobilize the joint. Joint motion is the first priority. Joint stiffness can be a significant problem in recovery from surgery.

Phase III: Strength Recovery phase (twelve weeks). At three months, the tendon repair should have significant strength to withstand active contraction. Although heavy lifting is to be avoided and contact activities are limited, most daily activities are allowed and progressing well in this stage. It can take eight to twelve months for the rotator cuff muscles to make a substantial recovery.

See Appendix C: Home Therapy Exercise Prescription

■ CHAPTER 6:
Frozen Shoulder (Adhesive Capsulitis)

◇ **Key Questions:**

- ❑ What is a frozen shoulder (adhesive capsulitis)?
- ❑ What causes the loss of motion and pain?
- ❑ How can frozen shoulder be treated?
- ❑ Is the injection safe, and will it hurt much?

◇ **Key additions:**

- ❑ A word on subtle frozen shoulder (posterior capsulitis)
- ❑ Home exercises required

What is a frozen shoulder (adhesive capsulitis)?

If the lining of **the socket becomes inflamed**, it can lead to loss of motion in the joint. It is this **loss of motion** in the shoulder joint—usually associated **with pain**—that is called a "frozen shoulder" (adhesive capsulitis).

Most patients do not remember injuring their shoulder before they notice the stiffness and pain. Often, a small incident like lifting a heavy grocery bag or suitcase may start the process, but it may take four to six weeks to develop the loss of motion and have pain.

The **loss of motion** can be subtle or profound. Rotation of the arm is usually the first motion affected. Often the first problem noticed is that a bra cannot be fastened or the back cannot be scratched. Often the ability to elevate the arm above shoulder level is affected as well.

Pain levels vary considerably depending on if the loss of motion is in its early stages or has advanced to its later stages. In general, the early stages are considerably more painful than the later stages. Pain interrupting sleep, sports, or work is often what drives a patient to seek help.

There are **two main types of frozen shoulder**. Some patients who get a frozen shoulder do not have an injury and do not have a systemic disease such as diabetes. This type is called **idiopathic** (or primary) frozen shoulder. Idiopathic means there is no known cause for the frozen shoulder.

Some patients get a frozen shoulder after an injury such as a rotator cuff tear or after shoulder surgery, or due to a systemic disease such as diabetes. This type is called **secondary** frozen shoulder. Secondary means it is the result of injury or a systemic disease. In many patients, the frozen shoulder is the first indication that there is a shoulder injury or a systemic disease.

Which type of frozen shoulder you have is important because the choice of treatment, the length of treatment, and the response to treatment can be very different between idiopathic and secondary frozen shoulder. In general, idiopathic frozen shoulder takes longer to treat than secondary frozen shoulder.

What causes the loss of motion and pain?

The early stages of frozen shoulder are caused by **inflammation**. The lining of the joint becomes inflamed, and this causes pain. Very early in the process, the loss of motion is mostly the result of pain from inflammation. This pain inhibits normal function of the muscles. Pain fibers in the joint send signals to the surrounding muscles that there is inflammation. Those muscles will involuntarily contract to prevent the joint from moving and causing further pain. This is a common protective reflex of the muscles to injury around any large joint.

In the later stages of frozen shoulder, the inflammation will begin to cause the lining of the joint to thicken with fibrosis tissue. This thick **scar tissue** replaces the normal elastic tissue. When this happens, motion is lost because the joint lining is scarred and contracted. (See Figure 6-1a.)

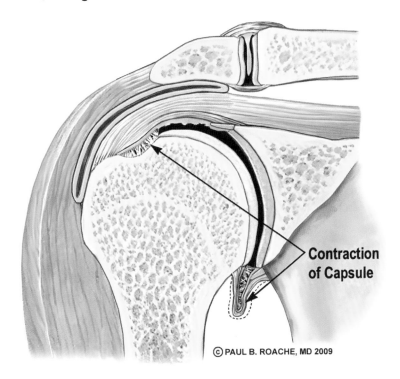

ADHESIVE CAPSULITIS

Figure 6-1a: The scarred and contracted lining of the joint in a frozen shoulder.

Normal motion usually preserves the elasticity of the lining of the joint and prevents fibrosis from thickening the joint lining. However, in frozen shoulder, normal motion is restricted, so fibrosis increases. Normal motion also maintains constant fluid movement in the joint. This fluid movement is very important for the nutrition and general health of the joint.

The **first goals of treatment are to interrupt the inflammation** and restore normal joint motion as soon as possible. This will reduce the fibrosis in the lining of the joint and restore normal fluid movement.

How can frozen shoulder be treated?

Using anti-inflammatory medicines interrupts inflammation. In order to deliver a concentrated dose of anti-inflammatory medicine to the joint, it is often best to have that medicine injected directly into the joint. This is the most effective way to relieve pain and interrupt inflammation.

When an injection is necessary, it should be performed as early as possible. This is because if it is performed in the very early stages of a frozen shoulder, it can quickly and completely restore normal motion. If it is performed in the later stages of a frozen shoulder, it is very effective at relieving pain, but restoring motion will be more difficult. When pain is reduced by the injection, it is easier for patients to perform the necessary stretching exercises and physical therapy that is required to restore motion. It is simply difficult to stretch the shoulder effectively when it hurts.

This is why, for the majority of patients, the most effective treatment is the injection followed by starting physical therapy and a home stretching program. Most patients in the early stages of a frozen shoulder will show significant improvement with treatment in three to six weeks.

In patients whom do not make satisfactory improvements towards restoring normal motion, I often order and MRI to look for a rotator cuff tear. Some patients will require a manipulation under anesthesia to get the shoulder moving. This is a stretching of the shoulder in the operating room while the patient is asleep and the muscles are relaxed. This is a very effective way to stretch the fibrosis/scar tissue and restore normal motion. Often at the same time, the arthroscope is used to release scar tissue and/or repair any tears in the rotator cuff. This is done as an outpatient procedure in a surgery center.

Is the injection safe, and will it hurt much?

The most common questions about the injection are about its safety and the discomfort of the injection. (See Chapter 7: Injections: Dispelling Common Misconceptions) The discomfort of the injection is generally very low. During a three-month period, patients in my practice were asked to rate their discomfort from the injection on a scale from zero to ten with ten being the highest pain. The average rating by my patients for this injection was two. In other words, most patients find the discomfort to be quite low.

The injections for most patients are very safe as well. A recent study indicated that four injections a year for up to two years could safely be performed. Overall, problems have rarely been reported in the scientific literature. In patients who have a compromised immune system, there is some concern about possible infection. However, only rare reports of this have been published. Over the last ten years, more than a thousand patients in my practice have received these injections. Only two patients have had any significant problems.

The injection takes less than twenty seconds to perform. Patients usually experience significant relief from pain within five to ten minutes after the injection. You can resume normal activities immediately after the injection the majority of the time. A few patients notice an achy pain the next day or two. This relieved by icing the shoulder. The medicine can stay active for three to four weeks.

In otherwise healthy patients, there is no known risk from the medicine. If you are an insulin-dependent diabetic with good control of your blood sugar, you can have the injection. However, you may have a short-term increase in your blood sugar, so you will need to supplement your diabetes routine. You should contact the doctor who treats your diabetes if there are any questions or problem.

• • •

A word on subtle frozen shoulder (posterior capsulitis)
The most common type of "frozen shoulder" I see in practice is a very subtle version called "posterior capsulitis" In basic terms, the problem of tightness is in the posterior inferior aspect of the capsule (socket). (See Figure 6-1b)

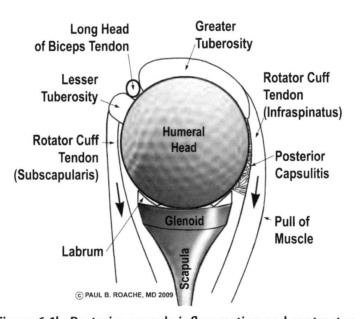

Figure 6-1b: Posterior capsule inflammation and contracture

It can be difficult for non-shoulder specialist to detect the problem. As such it can often be missed, and therefore untreated for a long period of time. The most sensitive way to detect a problem in the posterior capsule is to evaluate the internal rotation to the back. (Denoted as IRB) The difference from the affected side to the unaffected side can be as little as 2 inches. The good news is that once it has been detected, it is usually very treatable with anti-inflammatory injections and home exercises.

The most important treatment for these patients is the "Wall stretch" (see figures 6-4 and 6-5 below)

Home exercises required

The Wall stretch and the Table stretch are very important to make a recovery. It will take 6-8 weeks of daily work to see results. I tell patients it is like taffy that has hardened and must be worked constantly to soften and stretch. In essence this is true.

Shoulder Flexion Table Stretch
(See Figures 6-2 and 6-3)

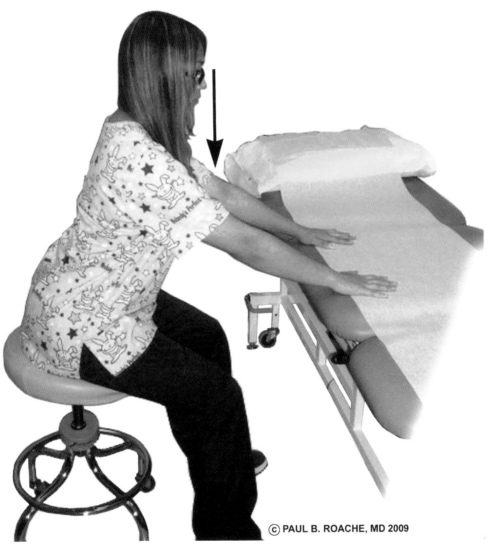

© PAUL B. ROACHE, MD 2009

Figure 6-2: Starting position for Flexion Table Stretch

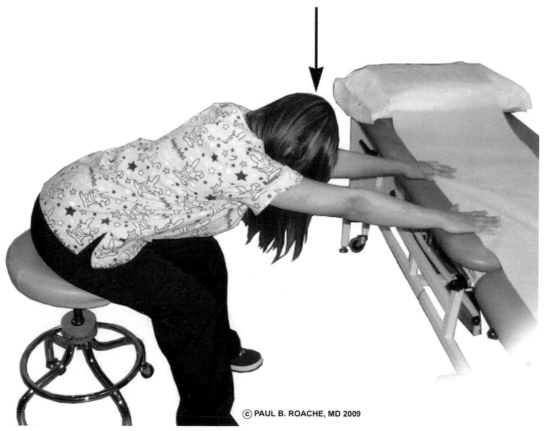

Figure 6-3: Finishing position for Flexion Table Stretch

1. Sit upright in a chair (preferably a chair with wheels).
2. Place both hands on a desktop or table in front of you.
3. Gently lean forward to stretch the shoulders. Keep shoulders square.
4. Hold for thirty seconds. Gradually work up to holding for two minutes over several weeks.
5. Perform five times daily.

Wall Stretch for Posterior Shoulder
(See Figure 6-4 and 6-5)

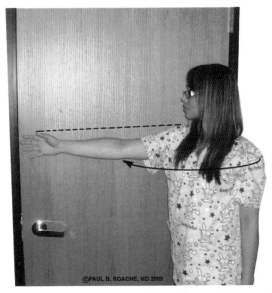

Figure 6-4: Starting position for Wall Stretch

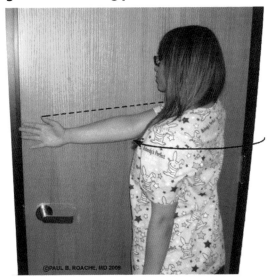

Figure 6-5: Finishing position for Wall Stretch

1. Stand with your shoulder against a wall or door.
2. Raise the arm to chest height. Try not to shrug the shoulder.
3. Keep the arm and shoulder against the wall; roll the body towards the arm.
4. Hold for thirty seconds. Gradually work up to holding for two minutes over several weeks.
5. Perform five times per day

Recommended Reading:

Mars, R. G., et al., "Intra-articular Corticosteroid Injection for Treatment of Idiopathic Adhesive Capsulitis of the Shoulder," *Hospital for Special Surgery Journal* 3 (2007): 202–207. (The authors presented strong evidence that early corticosteroid injections into the glenohumeral joint can have a profound benefit in shortening the recovery time.)

Cole, B. J., et al., "Injectable Corticosteroids in Modern Practice," *Journal of the American Academy of Orthopedic Surgeons* 13 (2005): 37–46. (The authors reviewed the orthopedic literature on the safety and efficacy of corticosteroid injections. The summary was that up to four injections a year for up to two years is safe and effective.)

CHAPTER 7:

Cortisone injections - Dispelling Common Misconceptions

◇ Key Questions:

- ❑ What are corticosteroids (cortisone)?
- ❑ How do corticosteroids work?
- ❑ How is the corticosteroid injected?
- ❑ Are corticosteroid injections painful?
- ❑ Do corticosteroids weaken bones?
- ❑ Do corticosteroids weaken tendons and ligaments?
- ❑ Is the effect temporary?
- ❑ Are there any risks?
- ❑ How often can injections be given?
- ❑ Can I do regular activities after the injection?

A word about common misconceptions:
Injections are safe powerful tools for treating and healing many shoulder problems. I have performed over one thousand shoulder injections and witnessed how they safely help many patients get well. Amazingly, patients who have never had injections have many misconceptions about this powerful treatment. These are the common questions these patients often ask.

What are corticosteroids?

Cortisone or my preferred choice kenalog, are in the family of drugs called corticosteroids. Corticosteroids are naturally occurring hormones made from cholesterol in the adrenal glands. They directly and indirectly affect the production of important enzymes in the body. In clinical practice, steroid injections are used for their **potent anti-inflammatory** effects. Corticosteroids are very different from the anabolic steroids used by athletes who have made recent headlines.

How do corticosteroids work?

Corticosteroids directly heal the inflammation in the area of the injection.

Normal cells in response to an injury usually produce inflammatory chemicals. Corticosteroids work on the cells to end the injury response. This stops the production of inflammatory chemicals. Often inflammation is present long after the initial injury, so healing inflammation can be permanent treatment. By healing the inflammatory process, the function of the shoulder will increase because there is less pain with movement. By reducing pain you will be able to exercise and strengthen your shoulder more effectively.

How is the corticosteroid injected?

Most of the time, they are injected with an anesthetic such as Lidocaine or Marcaine (similar to Novocain used by the dentist). The local anesthetic will have a noticeable effect within ten minutes. The pain should be reduced. Sometimes local nerves will also become numb temporarily. The steroid then soaks into the tissue; it will start working in the next several days. Occasionally it can take up to a week for a noticeable effect. The medicine is often working for up to thirty days.

Are corticosteroid injections painful?

Most patients have a low to moderate level of discomfort from the injection followed by relief from the anesthetic medicines. Most patients are pleasantly surprised. During a three-month period, patients in my practice were asked to rate their discomfort from the injection on a scale from zero to ten with ten being the highest pain. The average rating by my patients for this injection was two. In other words, most patients find the discomfort to be quite low. A few patients notice an achy pain the next day or two. This relieved by icing the shoulder. The medicine can stay active for three to four weeks.

Do corticosteroids weaken bones?

Although **oral** steroids can lead to bone loss, it does not seem to be an issue with judicious use of **injectable** corticosteroids.

Do corticosteroids weaken tendons and ligaments?

There is concern for patients who have rheumatoid arthritis, but in general, with judicious use, no current evidence suggests that harm is done to the tendons or ligaments.

Is the effect temporary?

The injection does not mask symptoms. And while the medicine itself is only working for up to thirty days, the effect can be long lasting. In fact, often it is curative. This is because often the pain and dysfunction of the shoulder is related to inflammation. So once the inflammation is healed, unless it is initiated again by injury, the problem is treated. **It is equivalent to hitting the restart button on your computer.**

Are there any risks?

Significant complications from steroid injections are rare (reported less than one in fifteen thousand). More commonly, patients will report soreness from the injection during the first day, but usually it is self-limiting. Occasionally, the skin will lose its normal pigment or local fat with atrophy. Allergic reactions to medicines are checked prior to the injection. Most people have been to the dentist, therefore, they know if Novocain style medications are safe for them.

In otherwise healthy patients, there is no known risk from the medicine. If you are an insulin-dependent diabetic with good control of your blood sugar, you can have the injection. However, you may have a short-term increase in your blood sugar, so you will need to supplement your diabetes routine. You should contact your doctor who treats your diabetes if there are any questions or problems.

How Often Can Injections Be Given?

A wide variety of opinions exist regarding the number of injections that are safe to receive. Most of the time, I limit them to three to four a year and no more frequently than every two months. (See recommended references at the end of chapter 6.)

Can I do regular activities after the injection?

The injection takes less than twenty seconds to perform. Patients usually experience significant relief from pain within five to ten minutes after the injection. You can resume normal activities immediately after the injection the majority of the time.

CHAPTER 8:

Shoulder Dislocations

◇ **Key Questions:**

- ❏ What is a dislocated shoulder?
- ❏ Why do shoulders dislocate or become loose?
- ❏ What are the treatment choices for a loose or dislocated shoulder?
- ❏ What type of surgery is performed to treat a dislocated shoulder?

What is a dislocated shoulder?

In Chapter 1, I discussed the key concept of the shoulder: **The shoulder is a ball-and-socket joint, but with a special socket.** When the **ball comes out of the socket**, this is called a **dislocation**. (See Figure 8-1a, 8-1b, and 8-1c)

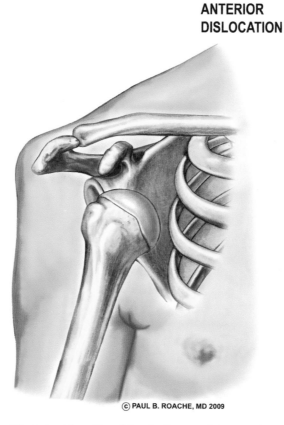

ANTERIOR DISLOCATION

© PAUL B. ROACHE, MD 2009

Fig 8-1a: The Shoulder ball out of the socket

BALL & SOCKET

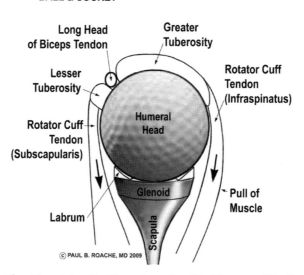

Long Head of Biceps Tendon

Greater Tuberosity

Lesser Tuberosity

Rotator Cuff Tendon (Infraspinatus)

Rotator Cuff Tendon (Subscapularis)

Humeral Head

Glenoid

Pull of Muscle

Labrum

Scapula

© PAUL B. ROACHE, MD 2009

Fig 8-1b: The Shoulder "ball-and-socket" is like a golf ball on a tee.

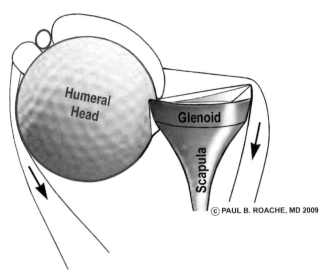

Figure 8-1c: The Shoulder ball out of the socket is like a golf ball off its tee

The socket is made of muscle, tendon, and ligaments. The ball can only come out of the socket if something tears in the socket and lets the ball dislocate. The something that tears is usually the Labrum and a key ligament in the front of the shoulder, an area called the Bankart Region. The labrum is tissue that rims the bony floor of the socket (glenoid). It is a soft type of cartilage deepens the socket. This helps keep the shoulder ball in the socket. This increased stability is very important for normal function of the shoulder. (See Figure 8-2a and 8-2b)

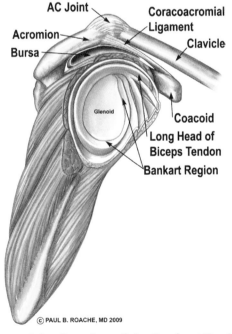

Figure 8-2a: Drawing of the Bankart Region

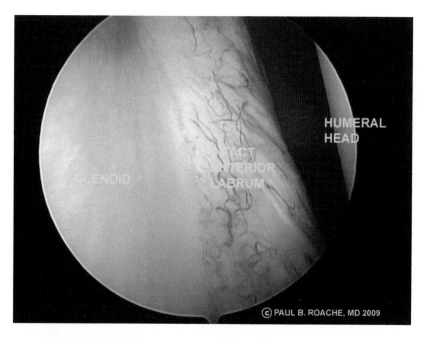

Figure8-2b: Arthroscopic picture of the Bankart Region

The tear of the labrum and ligament attachment to the socket in this region is called a **Bankart Lesion**. (See figure 8-3a and 8-3b)

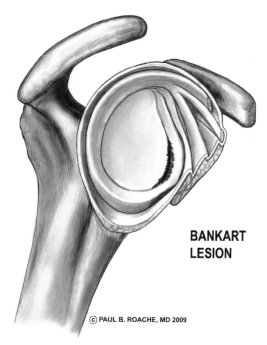

BANKART
LESION

Figure8-3a: Drawing of the Bankart Lesion

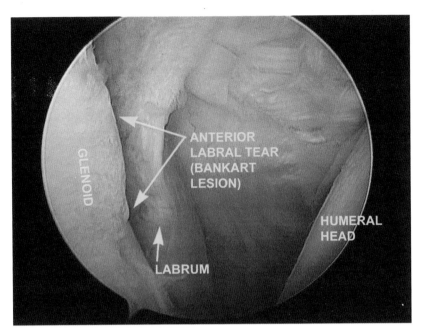

Figure8-3b: Arthroscopic Picture of the Bankart Lesion

The tear in the ligament rarely heals in its original position. Because of this, it does not function correctly and there is an increased risk of the dislocation reoccurring. Often surgical repair of the Bankart Lesion is required. (See figure 8-4a and 8-4b)

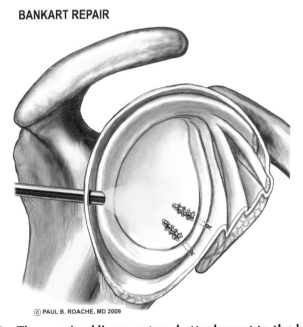

Fig 8-4a: The repaired ligament and attachment to the bone of the socket or "Bankart Repair"

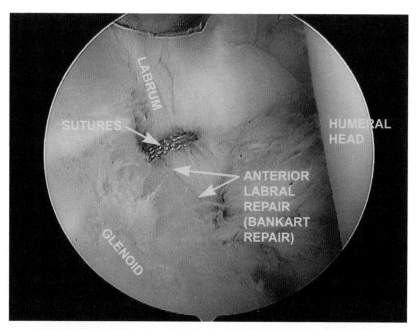

Fig 8-4b: Arthroscopic picture of the "Bankart Repair".

Why do shoulders dislocate or become loose?

The most common reason for a dislocation is a trauma to the shoulder from a fall. Some shoulders will become loose from repetitive motions performed as part of a sport or a job. Swimmers and gymnasts are good examples of people who can develop loose shoulders from repetitive stress on the socket. A loose shoulder is called an unstable shoulder.

Loose shoulders do not usually come all the way out of the joint. Typically, they move around in the socket, and the patient can feel that the ball is on the verge of coming out of the joint.

A very small number of patients have structural problems with the socket associated with how the bones formed prior to birth (called a congenital problem). These congenital problems set them up to have problems with a loose or dislocating shoulder.

In general, the younger you are when you have a dislocation, the higher the chance that the shoulder will keep coming out of the socket. In fact, if you are under thirty, very active, the chance of re-dislocating the shoulder is greater than 70 percent. If you are under twenty-five, the chance of re-dislocating is 98 percent. Because of the risk of re-dislocation in patients under thirty, it is often best to fix the torn ligament right after the first dislocation to prevent any further problems.

In patients over forty years old, the rate of re-dislocation is much lower, so often these patients can be treated without surgical repair of the ligament. However, these patients have an increased chance of tearing the rotator cuff tendons with a dislocation or a repeat dislocation. If the rotator cuff is torn from a dislocation, this is best treated with a surgical repair (see Chapter 2).

No matter what your age, each dislocation has a small, but very real risk of injuring the shoulder. First, nerves can be stretched, resulting in loss of sensation or weakness. Next, the bone of the glenoid and humerus can be fractured. Finally, the cartilage on the glenoid and the humeral head can be damaged. All of these injuries can have a serious long-term effect on how the shoulder can function.

What are the treatment choices for a loose or dislocated shoulder?

In patients who have developed a loose (unstable) shoulder from sports or work, we try to tighten the shoulder with physical therapy. If this is not successful, then surgical tightening is often necessary.

In patients who have a dislocated shoulder from a trauma, often I will surgically repair the ligament. This is best for a patient who is young enough to have a high chance of re-dislocating the shoulder or for an older patient who has not returned to full function after physical therapy.

<u>What type of surgery is performed to treat a dislocated shoulder?</u>

In general, **the surgery must reattach the ligament** in the front of the shoulder back to the bone in its normal position. This will restore the stability of the shoulder. (See Figures 8-4a and 8-4b above) This can be achieved either using the arthroscope or through the traditional open surgery. (See WebRX: "Repair of detached labrum" or "Bankart repair.")
I perform most of these as arthroscopic repairs, with very good results. However, there are certain patients and types of problems that are more successfully treated with the traditional open surgery.

Recommended Reading

Matsen III, F. A., Titelman, R. M., Lippitt, S. B., Rockwood, C. A., and Wirth, M. A., "Glenohumeral Instability," in *The Shoulder*, 3rd edition, ed., C. A. Rockwood, F. A. Matsen III, M. A. Wirth, and S. B. Lippitt (Philadelphia, PA: Saunders, 2004), 655-790.

Neer II, C. S., and Foster, C. R., "Inferior Capsular Shift for Involuntary Inferior and Multidirectional Instability of the Shoulder: A Preliminary Report," *Journal of Bone and Joint Surgeons*, American edition 62, 6 (1980): 897-908.

CHAPTER 9:

SLAP Tears and Biceps Tendon Injuries

◇ **Key Questions:**

- ❑ What does SLAP stand for?
- ❑ What is the function of the SLAP region?
- ❑ How do you know you have a SLAP injury?
- ❑ How do you treat SLAP tears?

What does SLAP stand for?

The labrum is soft tissue that rims the bony floor of the shoulder socket. SLAP stands for **Superior Labrum Anterior Posterior**. This refers to the labrum in the upper (superior) region of the shoulder socket. It includes the labrum in the front (anterior) and the back (posterior) of the region. Hence, the acronym for the region: **S**uperior **L**abrum **A**nterior **P**osterior. (See figure 9-1)

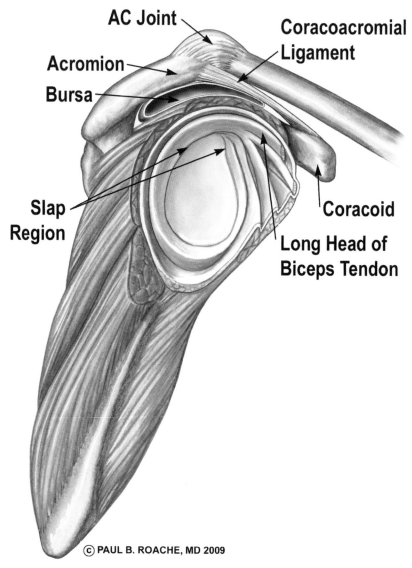

AC Joint

Coracoacromial
Ligament

Acromion

Bursa

Slap
Region

Coracoid

Long Head of
Biceps Tendon

© PAUL B. ROACHE, MD 2009

Figure 9-1: The SLAP Region of the Shoulder

What is the function of the SLAP region?

The labrum is tissue that rims the bony floor of the socket (glenoid). It is a soft type of cartilage deepens the socket. This helps keep the shoulder ball in the socket. This increased stability is very important for normal function of the shoulder. A tendon from the biceps attaches to the top of the labrum and tensions the labrum. This increases the stability provided from the labrum. This is important for stabilizing the shoulder when the arm is at shoulder level or higher. The biceps tendon can be injured with the labrum or by itself (See Figure 9-2.)

SLAP TEAR

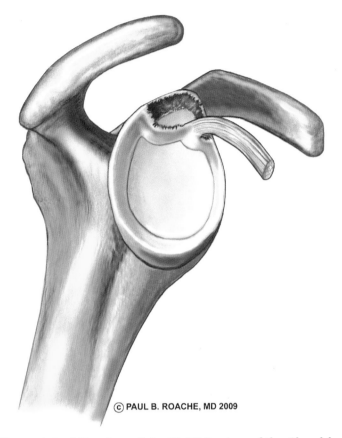

© PAUL B. ROACHE, MD 2009

Figure 9-2; A Tearing of the SLAP Region of the Shoulder

How do you know you have a SLAP injury?

The most common symptom is **pain with overhead activities**. Sometimes patients report "clunking" in the shoulder with activities. But neither is very specific. MRI has proven to be unreliable for identifying SLAP tears. The most important part of diagnosing a SLAP injury is the examination from a shoulder specialist. The second most important part of diagnosing a SLAP injury is an intra-articular injection with Lidocaine. The injection confirms that the pain is coming from the SLAP injury.

Note:
While MRI is not reliable for demonstrating SLAP injuries, it is useful for assessing the shoulder for associated injuries of the rotator cuff.

How do you treat SLAP tears?

As with most shoulder injuries, inflammation can be a significant source of pain and dysfunction with SLAP injuries. A significant tear of the labrum or biceps tendon can be pinched in the joint and continue causing pain and dysfunction. The intra-articular injection with Lidocaine is usually combined with a powerful anti-inflammatory like Cortisone. If the inflammation is the major cause of the problem, then the injection can be curative. If the tear is the major cause of the problem, then the problem will return. However, good relief from an injection, even if temporary, confirms that surgical treatment can be successful. The surgical treatment involves trimming small tears and repairing large tears. (See Figure 9-3.)

REPAIR OF SLAP TEAR

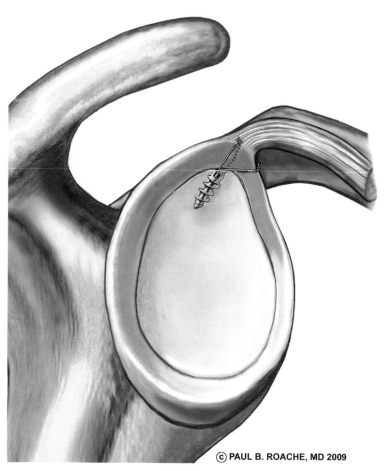

© PAUL B. ROACHE, MD 2009

Figure 9-3: The Repair of a SLAP tear

Special Category of SLAP injuries

SLAP tear with a paralabral cyst:
A cyst can form from the **joint fluid that leaks out of the joint** from a SLAP tear. It can push the thin capsule into a balloon like cyst. These can be quite large. Sometimes they are big enough that they push into the muscle and cause pain. If they are large enough, they can even push onto the suprascapular nerve and cause weakness in the external rotators of the rotator cuff. (See Figure 9-4.)

PARALABRAL CYST WITH SUPRASCAPULAR NERVE

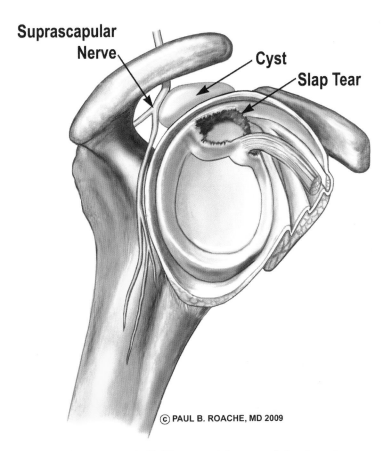

Figure 9-4: A SLAP tear with a paralabral cyst

The treatment for cysts that are causing symptoms or weakness is surgical, involving treatment of the SLAP and often a drainage or removal of the cyst.

CHAPTER 10

Neck Problems and Nerve Problems of the Shoulder

◇ **Key questions:**
- ❑ Why does my neck hurt with my shoulder injury?
- ❑ Can my neck cause problems in my shoulder?
- ❑ How do nerve problems cause shoulder problems?

Why does my neck hurt with my shoulder injury?
The supporting muscles of the shoulder blade can be affected by a shoulder injury. These muscles can be stretched or overworked to compensate for the injury. The muscles that attach the shoulder blade to the neck are the most commonly affected.

Patients will often have neck pain or spasms in those muscles. Medication, ice, and/or heat can help in the short run. The long-term solution is to heal the shoulder injury. (See Chapter 1 and Figure 10-1.)

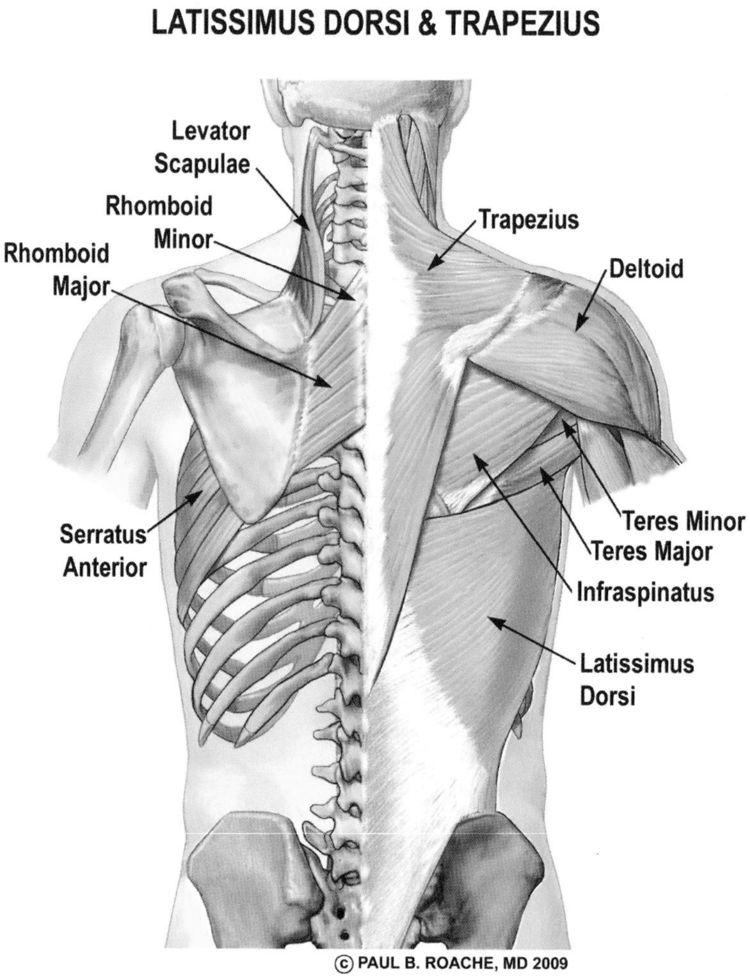

LATISSIMUS DORSI & TRAPEZIUS

Levator Scapulae

Rhomboid Minor

Rhomboid Major

Trapezius

Deltoid

Serratus Anterior

Teres Minor

Teres Major

Infraspinatus

Latissimus Dorsi

© PAUL B. ROACHE, MD 2009

Figure 10-1: Muscles of the shoulder blade and neck

Can my neck cause problems in my shoulder?

This is a relatively complicated topic. The simple answer is yes. Muscles attaching to the neck and nerves that come from the neck can often cause shoulder pain and dysfunction. The most common situation is pain in the shoulder that is coming from irritation of the nerves in the neck. In simple terms, nerves are the body's version of wire, and carry the electrical signals from the brain that let the muscles perform their action. They also carry the signals of pain, and send signals of position to the brain. In the shoulder, six nerve roots come from the neck. Five of these combine into a nerve center for the shoulder and arm called the brachial plexus. The brachial plexus then gives off multiple nerves that operate the muscles of the shoulder and give sensation to the region. The two most important nerves to the shoulder are the suprascapular nerve and the axillary nerve. (See Figure 10-2)

What can make this topic complicated is finding the cause of the irritation to the nerves. This can often involve testing by a neurologist, and an MRI. Fortunately, for most patients, the irritation is transient, and they will not need a neurologist to find the irritation to the nerves.

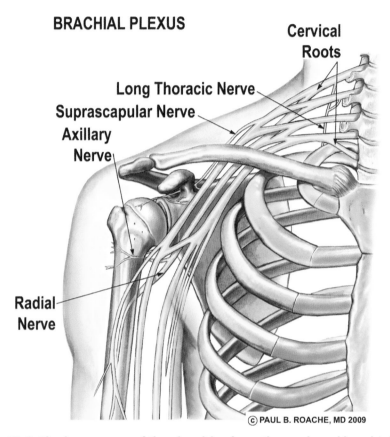

BRACHIAL PLEXUS

Cervical Roots

Long Thoracic Nerve

Suprascapular Nerve

Axillary Nerve

Radial Nerve

© PAUL B. ROACHE, MD 2009

Figure 10-2: The key nerves of the shoulder from the neck and brachial plexus

How do nerve problems cause shoulder problems?

This too can be a relatively complicate topic. It depends if the nerve problem is coming from the neck, the collection of nerves below the collarbone (brachial plexus), or the specific nerves that operate the shoulder (axillary, suprascapular, long thoracic, and dorsal scapular).

The most common nerve problem of the shoulder comes from the irritation of the nerves that exit from the neck. This frequently shows up as shoulder pain and or weakness. Frequently the pain is described as "burning" pain. Often there is pain that travels down the arm or to the shoulder blade. Sometimes patients will report numbness (pins and needle sensation) in the arm, forearm, or hand. The key to treating this nerve problem is to diagnose the cause of the irritation of the nerves coming from the neck.

Less commonly, the specific nerves that operate the shoulder can be injured. This can happen with a variety of traumas to the shoulder. The most common is an injury to the axillary nerve when the shoulder dislocates. The axillary nerve operates the large deltoid muscle of the shoulder and one muscle in the rotator cuff. Most of these injuries will make a full recovery with time. But it can take many months.

Least common are injuries to the collection of nerves below the collarbone (the brachial plexus). These nerves can be stretched by a trauma, or inflammation or a virus can affect them. The diagnosis of these nerve injuries requires a thorough evaluation by a neurologist. Treatment can be determined after the evaluation by the neurologist. Frequently, the neurologist will test how the muscles are receiving the nerve impulse and how the nerves are carrying the impulse. This testing is called a "Nerve conduction study and electromyography" (NCS/EMG).

CHAPTER 11:

Clavicle Fractures (collarbone fractures)

◇ **Key Questions:**

- ❑ How does the clavicle get broken?
- ❑ When is surgery needed?
- ❑ Why are plates and screws used in surgery?
- ❑ What is the role of the clavicle?

How does the collarbone get broken?

A direct fall on to the shoulder is the most common way to break the collarbone. Most fractures of the collarbone will heal well on their own. However, there are certain types of fractures that will need surgery to heal well. (See Figure 11-1.)

FRACTURED CLAVICLE

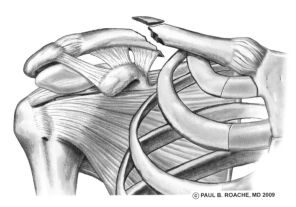

© PAUL B. ROACHE, MD 2009

Figure 11-1: Fracture of the collarbone or clavicle

When is surgery needed?

Immediate surgery is needed when there is a break in the skin over the fracture, or the edge of the fracture is putting pressure on the skin, or there are nerve symptoms from pressure caused by the fracture. Fortunately, this is very uncommon.

More commonly, surgery is needed when the gap between the pieces is too large, or the overlap of the pieces is too great. If the gap between pieces is too large, the fracture may take a very long time to heal or not heal at all. Rather than investing four to six months of time to see if a fracture will heal, it is more predictable to have surgery. That is because at surgery, the gap is reduced and the pieces of the fracture are held together with a plate and screws. This aids the body in efficiently completing the healing process.

If the overlap of the pieces is too great, the fracture may heal in a position that makes the collarbone much shorter. This can prevent the shoulder from functioning normally. First, it can affect the range of motion of the shoulder. Second, it can affect the strength of the shoulder. In some cases of overlap, the pieces heal and create a larger mass of bone. This larger mass of bone can push on the important nerves below the collarbone. These nerves operate the muscles and sensations of the shoulder, arm, and hand. Normally, the collarbone protects these nerves. But if the mass of bone is too large, the nerves can be injured. (See Chapter 10.)

Occasionally, an athlete will have surgery on a fracture expected to heal well. This is done to ensure that they return to their sport as quickly as possible. High-level cyclists are the most likely to request this. This is a very special situation and requires an in-depth evaluation of the athlete's situation, because it carries some extra risks. Consult your shoulder specialist for more information.

Why are plates and screws used in surgery?

Today, the technology for fixing these fractures is very good. Special plates shaped to match the collarbone have improved the results of surgical treatment greatly. These plates and screws are the strongest way to hold the pieces of the fracture together. By holding the pieces together, the body can efficiently go through the healing process. Today's plates are very smooth and thin. They are rarely felt under the skin, and rarely need to be removed after the healing. (See Figure 11-2.)

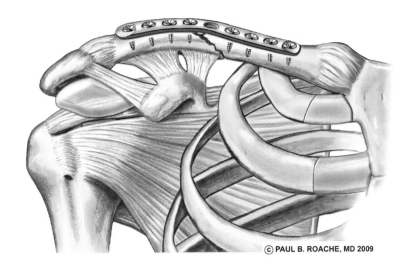

© PAUL B. ROACHE, MD 2009

CLAVICULAR REPAIR
Figure 11-2: Clavicle Fracture repair with plate and screws

What is the role of the clavicle?

The clavicle is the only bone connecting the shoulder blade and the arm to the central skeleton. In essence, the clavicle is like a suspension bridge between the spines central skeleton and the shoulder blade (scapula) and arm. The shoulder blade and arm are actually suspended from the distal end of the clavicle. The ends of the clavicle are held in place by very strong ligaments. The inside end of the clavicle (medial) creates the Sternoclavicular joint (SC joint) at the central skeleton(the Sternum). The outside end (lateral or distal) creates the Acromioclavicular joint (AC Joint). (See Figure 11-3)

Injuries to the Clavicle and or the AC joint will result in a disruption of the connection between the central skeleton and shoulder blade/arm. This results in a loss of position of the shoulder blade/arm. When this happens the shoulder blade/arm are dropping down away from the clavicle. Muscles attached to the clavicle will now pull unopposed by the weight of the shoulder blade/arm. The result of the arm dropping down and away and the muscles pulling the clavicle up creates the typical deformities seen with clavicle fractures and AC joint injuries.

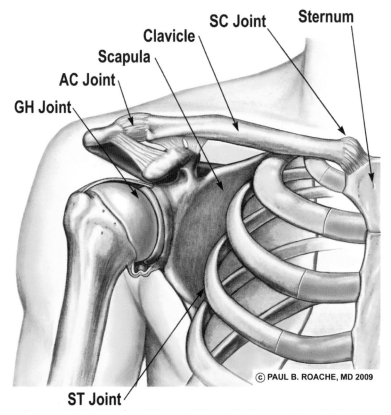

Figure 11-3: The clavicle and the SC joint and the AC joint

CHAPTER 12:

Shoulder Separations/AC Joint Injuries

◇ **Key Questions:**

- ❑ What is a shoulder separation?
- ❑ Will they heal on their own?
- ❑ When is surgery needed?
- ❑ What is the role of the clavicle?

What is a shoulder separation?

The collarbone is connected to the shoulder blade at the top of the shoulder blade. This region is called the acromion. The joint between the collarbone and the acromion is called the **AC joint (acromioclavicular joint).** Three sets of important ligaments hold the AC joint together. When part or all of these ligaments are injured, this is called a **shoulder separation.** This most commonly occurs by a direct fall onto the shoulder. (See Figures 12-1 and 12-2.)

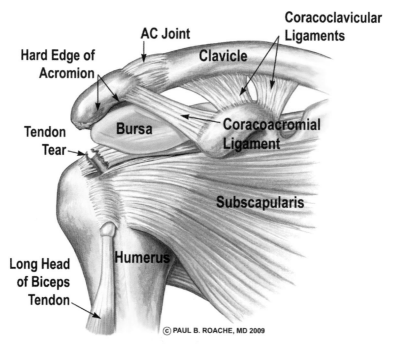

Figure 12-1: **Normal AC joint and its ligaments**

These injuries occur in **four degrees** of severity.

Grade 1: injury to only the ligaments at the AC joint itself.

Grade 2: injury to the ligaments of the AC joint and a partial injury to the CC ligaments. There is a partial displacement of the collarbone upwardly.

Grade 3: injury to both sets of ligaments. There is a complete displacement of the collarbone upwardly.

Grade 4+: injury to both sets of ligaments. There is a complete displacement of the collarbone through the trapezius muscle and it is stuck up and behind the AC joint. Or it could even be displaced below and in front of the AC joint.

Grade 1 and 2 are the most common AC joint injuries.

GRADE 3 INJURY

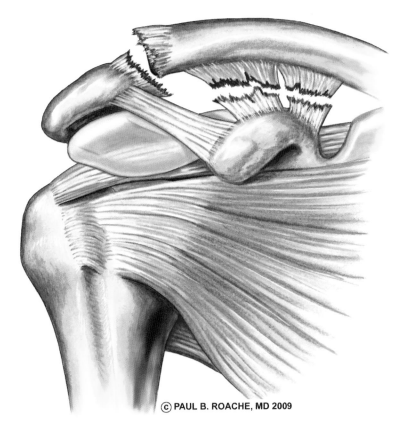

© PAUL B. ROACHE, MD 2009

Figure 12-2; Injured AC joint and its torn ligaments

Will they heal on their own?

Fortunately, most of the injuries from Grade 1 to 3 will heal on their own. This is because the ligaments can generate scar tissue. This scar tissue can hold the torn ligaments together. This can restore the normal function to the ligaments that were torn. Once the ligaments are back to normal function, the shoulder will return to normal function.

When is surgery needed?

In certain cases, the function of the shoulder can be affected by a shoulder separation. Usually, surgery is reserved for injuries that involve all three sets of ligaments (Grade 3), in patients who put very high demands on their shoulders. For example, a quarterback with a Grade 3 injury is a patient who puts high demand on his shoulder and may need surgery. A recreational tennis player with a Grade 3 injury usually does not need surgery. All patients with Grade 4 injuries or higher will need surgery. The type of surgery performed varies with the situation and the severity of the injury.

What is the role of the clavicle?
The clavicle is the only bone connecting the shoulder blade and the arm to the central skeleton. In essence, the clavicle is like a suspension bridge between the spines central skeleton and the shoulder blade (scapula) and arm. The shoulder blade and arm are actually suspended from the distal end of the clavicle. The ends of the clavicle are held in place by very strong ligaments. The inside end of the clavicle (medial) creates the Sternoclavicular joint (SC joint) at the central skeleton(the Sternum). The outside end (lateral or distal) creates the Acromioclavicular joint (AC Joint). (See Figure 12-3)

Injuries to the Clavicle and or the AC joint will result in a disruption of the connection between the central skeleton and shoulder blade/arm. This results in a loss of position of the shoulder blade/arm. When this happens the shoulder blade/arm are dropping down away from the clavicle. Muscles attached to the clavicle will now pull unopposed by the weight of the shoulder blade/arm. The result of the arm dropping down and away and the muscles pulling the clavicle up creates the typical deformities seen with clavicle fractures and AC joint injuries.

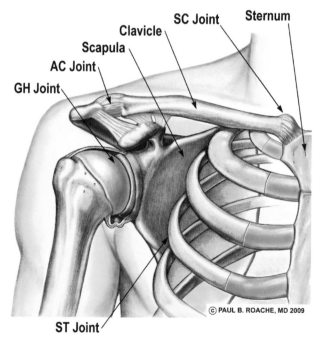

Figure 12-3: The clavicle and the SC joint and the AC joint

■ CHAPTER 13:

Shoulder Fractures

◇ Key Questions:

- ❑ What parts of the shoulder are most commonly fractured?
- ❑ Which fractures will heal without surgery?
- ❑ When surgery is needed, what will be done?

What parts of the shoulder are most commonly fractured?

While any bone in the shoulder can be fractured, the bone most commonly fractured is the clavicle (see Chapter 11). The next most common shoulder bone fractured is the ball (proximal humerus). The least common shoulder bone fractured is the shoulder blade (scapula).

When the bone of the proximal humerus (ball) breaks, **there are four things that are important to assess.**

<u>First</u>, **which part or parts of the bone have been injured?** (See Figure 13-1)

PROXIMAL HUMERUS

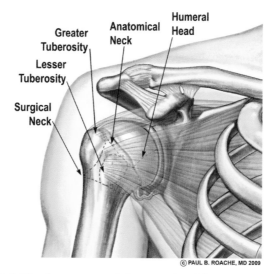

Figure 13-1: The key parts of the proximal humerus to evaluate

Second, are those injured parts displaced from their normal position?

Third, do any of the injured parts have rotator cuff tendons attached? (See Figure 13-2)

FRACTURED GREATER TUBEROSITY
WITH ROTATOR CUFF TENDON

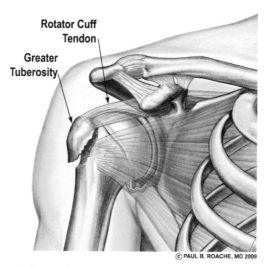

Figure 13-2: Greater Tuberosity fracture displaced by the pull of the rotator cuff

<u>Fourth,</u> is there a fracture that involves the joint surface? (See Figure 13-3)

ANATOMICAL NECK FRACTURE

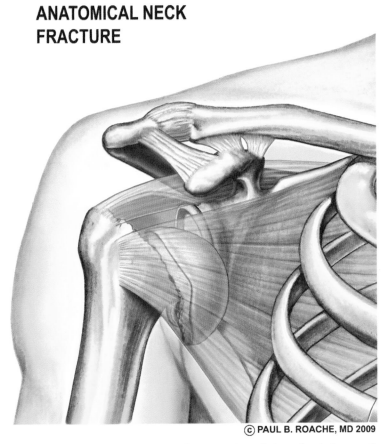

© PAUL B. ROACHE, MD 2009

Figure 13-3: Proximal Humerus fracture involving the joint surface

The most common of these fractures is at the junction of the humeral shaft with the ball. This area is called the surgical neck. Fractures of the surgical neck can heal on their own if they are not displaced. (See Figure 13-4)

SURGICAL NECK FRACTURE OF HUMERUS

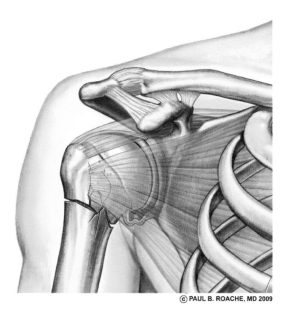

© PAUL B. ROACHE, MD 2009

Figure 13-4: Proximal Humerus fracture at the surgical neck

Which fractures will heal without surgery?

In general, if the fracture has not displaced from its normal position or is minimally displaced, the fracture can be treated in a sling, and it will heal on its own. The one exception to this is for elderly patients, who have fractured a hip or leg and the shoulder. In this case, surgery for the shoulder fracture may be needed to help them get out of bed and use a walker or crutch.

When surgery is needed, what will be done?

Three types of fractures in the shoulder usually need surgery. First is a fracture of the bone to which the rotator cuff tendons attach (greater or lesser tuberosity). When these fractures are displaced, the rotator cuff function is in jeopardy. (See Figure 13-2) These are usually treated by sewing the piece or pieces back in position. Some of these can be performed with arthroscopic assistance. Sometimes these are fixed with pins or a screw. (See Figure 13-5.)

REPAIR OF GREATER TUBEROSITY

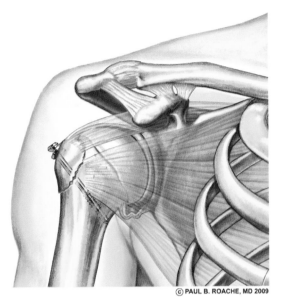

© PAUL B. ROACHE, MD 2009

Figure 13-5: The fracture of the Greater Tuberosity reduced and fixed with a screw

<u>Second</u> is a displaced fracture of the surgical neck (see Figure 13-4). If the humeral shaft and ball are out of alignment or not in at least 50 percent contact, the bone may heal in a bad position or not heal at all. These are usually fixed with a plate and screws or pins. (See Figure 13-6.)

REPAIR OF SURGICAL NECK FRACTURE

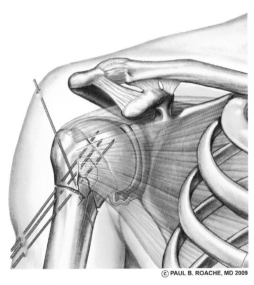

© PAUL B. ROACHE, MD 2009

Figure 13-6: The fracture of the surgical neck fixed with pins

Third is a fracture that displaces the joint surface. (See Figure 13-3) A fracture of the ball (humeral head) that is displaced can severely affect how the shoulder works and can lead to deterioration of the joint. Some of these fractures can be fixed with a plate and screws. Some require a partial joint replacement. (See Figure 13-7)

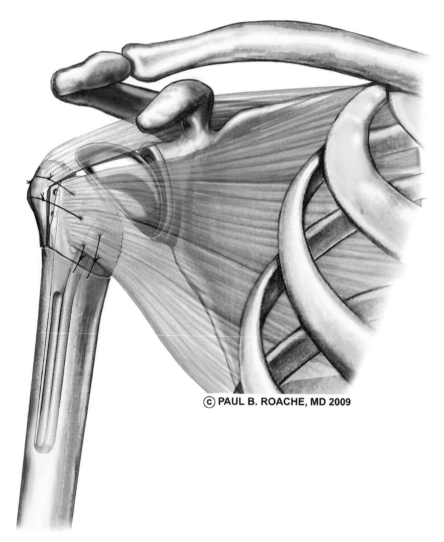

© PAUL B. ROACHE, MD 2009

Figure 13-7: Partial joint replacement for displaced fracture of the joint surface

CHAPTER 14

Shoulder Arthritis

◇ Key Questions:

- ❑ What is arthritis?
- ❑ How can it be treated?
- ❑ When should I consider a shoulder replacement?
- ❑ What can I expect from a shoulder replacement?

What is arthritis?

The bone in joints is lined with a smooth tissue that helps the bones glide over each other and cushions the bones. This is called cartilage. **When the cartilage is worn away, the bones no longer glide smoothly over each other, and they have lost their cushion. This is called arthritis.** It is also called degenerative joint disease. It is commonly associated with pain and joint dysfunction. The large joints, the hip and knee, commonly develop arthritis as patients age. The shoulder develops arthritis, but at a lower rate than the hip or the knee. Pain and inability to sleep from that pain are the most common reasons patients go to the shoulder surgeon when they have shoulder arthritis. (See Figure 14-1.)

SHOULDER ARTHRITIS

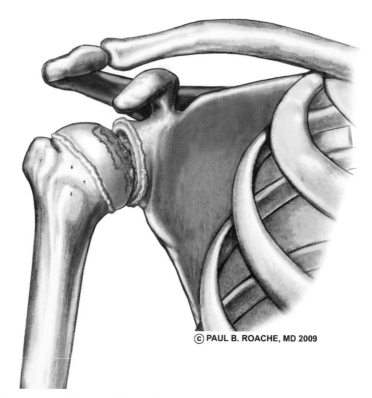

© PAUL B. ROACHE, MD 2009

Figure 14-1:The roughened joint surface of Shoulder arthritis

How can it be treated?
In the early stages, shoulder arthritis can be significantly treated with oral medications like Ibuprofen (Motrin), activity modifications, and exercise. In the later stages, injections of Cortisone into the joint can be very effective in treating the inflammation and pain of the arthritis.

When should I consider a shoulder replacement?
When the pain can no longer be treated with medicines or injections, it is time to consider having the joint replaced. This involves removing the rough arthritic surface of the ball and socket and replacing them a smooth metal and plastic surface. (See Figure 14-2.)

TOTAL SHOULDER REPLACEMENT

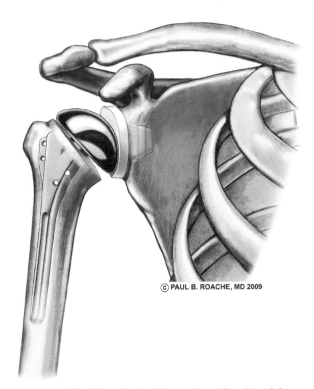

© PAUL B. ROACHE, MD 2009

Figure 14-2: The Metal ball and plastic socket of a shoulder replacement

What can I expect from a shoulder replacement?

Shoulder replacements are excellent at relieving the shoulder pain that comes from arthritis. In most patients, motion is also improved. They are as successful as hip and knee replacements. The surgery for a shoulder replacement requires usually an overnight stay in the hospital. Often, the anesthesiologist will insert medicine to numb the nerves of the shoulder and prevent pain. This is called a regional anesthetic (interscalene or supraclavicular block). In some cases, a thin tube (like those used for epidural anesthesia) is inserted under ultrasound guidance next to the nerves of the shoulder. The anesthesiologist then attaches a small pump that drips anesthetic to keep the nerves numb. This can prevent any pain for several days. Usually, you will be in a sling for three to six weeks.

Pendulum exercises only are permitted during this time. The surgery requires detaching the front of the rotator cuff to get into the joint (subscapularis tendon). It is reattached at the end of surgery. This is essentially like a rotator cuff repair. Like a rotator cuff repair, it must be protected for three to six weeks, so it can start to heal and not come loose. This is why exercises are limited for three to six weeks after surgery.

• • •

Special Category of Shoulder Replacement.
Arthritis that develops as a result of a very large rotator cuff tear can also cause significant pain and dysfunction. Some patients are unable to life their arm high enough to even comb their hair because the rotator cuff is so torn that it is not functioning. These patients can be treated with a special type of shoulder replacement called **the reverse ball-and-socket**. It is designed to allow patients to lift their arm above their shoulder. It does so by using the deltoid to compensate for the ineffective rotator cuff. It is able to do so because the ball is reversed and placed on the glenoid and the socket is placed on the proximal humerus. When the deltoid contracts it rotates the socket around the ball.
(See Figure 14-3)

REVERSE BALL & SOCKET

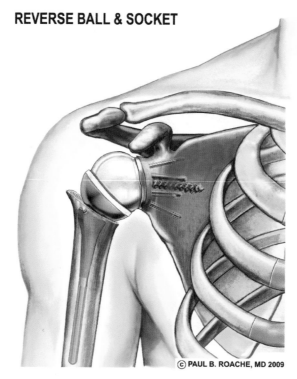

© PAUL B. ROACHE, MD 2009

Figure 14-3: The reverse ball-and-socket prosthesis

Note: The reverse ball-and-socket prosthesis has been used successfully for many years in Europe. My first experience with it was in 1999 while visiting Zurich. It has been in use in the United States for several years. It provides certain patients with a treatment than can have dramatic benefits, but it also has approximately a 20 percent complication rate. You should consult your shoulder surgeon for further information.

■ CHAPTER 15:
Chiropractic Care in Shoulder Injuries

By Richard L. Brent, DC

Overview:
A Doctor of Chiropractic Medicine is trained in musculoskeletal health and disease from a very different perspective than a Shoulder Surgeon. Our training empha-sizes Spinal alignment and the effects of misalignment that play a role in pain and dysfunction in the musculoskeletal system. Soft tissue treatments as well as direct spinal alignment may be called for to restore balance in the musculoskeletal tissues of a shoulder with dysfunction.

My Role in treating Rotator Cuff Injuries:
The objective is to restore balance, function and proper range of motion of the shoulder joint. A shoulder impaired by a Rotator Cuff Injury will often transfer the workload to the surrounding muscles of the shoulder girdle. This can lead to spinal misalignment, muscle spasm, and cervical nerve root irritation. My role is to treat the cascade of dysfunction that accompanies a Rotator Cuff injury. By doing so I effectively find out which patients will be able heal and which patients will need injection therapy or surgical treatment.

In patients who require surgical care I can assist in the physical preparation for surgery. After Surgery patients can also have a cascade of problems related to the healing and recovery from surgery. Chiropractic care can be a significant adjunct in the recovery process.

How do I as a Chiropractor treat Shoulder pain and injuries?

1. A proper exam is performed to determine the nature of the dysfunction, the location of pain and possible causes. This may include but not limited to the surrounding areas of the chest, arm, neck and back.
2. Typical treatment would involve managing the muscles and soft tissues of the shoulder to restore range of motion (ROM), proper function, and strength with balance of all the shoulder muscles. This treatment is often implemented prior to surgery while not affecting the area of surgical repair. This will help prepare a patient for postoperative recovery. Clearly, synergy with the Orthopedic Surgeon is most affective for the patient's care.
3. Management of soft tissue may include, Ultra-sound, E-stim, ice, heat, myofacial release techniques, trigger point therapy and specific joint mobilization to breakup fibrous adhesions, scar tissue, and remove muscle spasm. The objective is to restore balance, function and proper range of motion of the shoulder joint.
4. Specific rehabilitation exercises to restore strength, balance and ROM are incorporated into the treatment. These exercises are performed at the office and often become part of a patient's daily activities to maintain the strength and integrity of the shoulder joint.

The shoulder joint can have many injuries. Some examples that Chiropractors treat involve frozen shoulder, sprain/strains, and Rotator Cuff injuries. Further, subacromial and sub-deltoid bursitis can also be the cause of shoulder tenderness and restriction.

Will the treatment involve other areas of the body other than the shoulder?

Yes, associated muscles are often involved in the shoulder dysfunction and can be as important as treating the shoulder region itself. These may include the arm muscles; biceps, triceps, and deltoids, the chest muscles, neck and upper back muscles which include but not limited to Pectoralis major, Sternocleidomastoid, Trapezius, Rhomboid, and Levator scapula.

Does Chiropractic Care adjust or mobilize the neck and back when treating shoulder problems?

Yes. The neck and back joint immobility, often called subluxations, may often cause or develop as a result of shoulder pain and dysfunction. Maintaining joint mobility is imperative for the proper function of the muscles of the neck, shoulder and back.

Richard L. Brent, D.C., QME
2535 Mission St.
San Francisco, CA 94110
Ph: 415-826-1000
Fx: 415-826-0999
http://missionchiro.com

■ CHAPTER 16:
Yoga for the Shoulder: Working with Injury

By Jason Crandell   *www.jasonyoga.com*

Unlike various modalities that focus on the injury present, yoga seeks to address the entire body, the nervous system and the mind. While a well-guided yoga practitioner can target various physical ailments and work specifically to rehabilitate them, the focus of a yoga practice is always much broader than the specific injury being addressed. Yoga seeks to facilitate harmony between the body, breath, mind, and—depending on one's philosophical persuasion—the spirit. This is the case if one has adhesive capsulitis, a rotator complication, or no shoulder complications at all. Simply stated, the goal of yoga—for those with and without shoulder complications alike—is the same: To cultivate a state of clarity, cohesion, and awareness in all of the layers of one's self. Shoulder injuries, however, can make this pursuit more complicated for two reasons.

To begin with, it is difficult to focus on anything other than the pain when you are confronted with a shoulder injury. Feeling the whole body and cultivating a sense of wellbeing is difficult when pain hijacks your attention and makes you feel rotten. To make matters more challenging, nearly everyone gets frustrated and encounters fear when they have an injury. This scenario compounds as the days, weeks—and, sometimes, months and years—tick by. Often, people with injuries—especially chronic injuries—perceive their entire body as faulty and problematic. As the psychological and emotional weight of an injury mounts, many become *less* inclined to pursue the processes that may lead to healing because they no longer like the body that they inhabit—for some, the body has become an unwelcome necessity at best, or a hostile enemy at worst. Others adapt to their pain by pushing through the symptoms, which can make matters worse.

The second hurdle for injured practitioners is modifying the poses in such a way that the shoulder pain is decreased—or, at least, not made worse. Shoulder modifications often require individualized attention and an exhaustive list is not possible in this medium. Most importantly, you will see how a smart, consistent yoga practice fosters the physical, mental and emotional environment for health and healing.

• • •

New start

At first glance, practicing yoga with a rotator cuff injury or adhesive capsulitis can seem quite difficult. For some experienced students, working with these shoulder complications can alter the practice so substantially that they'd rather sit on the sidelines reciting "give me down dog, chatturanga, and handstand, or give me nothing at all." For less experienced practitioners, the shear discomfort and complexity of these shoulder challenges—and, of course, the fear that accompanies them—is so overwhelming that they don't know where to begin.

While the challenges are real and substantial—from the pain to the limitation in mobility, strength, and comfort—sustaining a thorough, satisfying yoga practice while injured is not only possible, but also instrumental in sustaining the physical and mental state conducive to healing.

Consider the most important issue regarding yoga and local pain of any sort: The entire body does not need to suffer because one area of the body has a limitation or is encountering pain. All too often, people allow the injury in a local area to control the behavior of the entire body. This is like deciding not to brush all of your teeth because one tooth has a cavity.

I remember talking to a student with adhesive capsulitis about how their practice was going. They paused for a long-time and, somewhat ashamed, said that they weren't able to practice yoga because of the injury. The student followed by saying, "you know, I can't even do down-dog." I asked her how her feet, legs and knees were doing and she said they were fine. Then I asked how her hips, spine, and abs were doing. Again, they were fine. A long-pause ensued and I asked her why she was letting the inability to do down-dog like she was used to doing it interfere with her ability to practice nearly everything else. The answer was that she was scared of the injury, frustrated with her body and annoyed with her injury—and, more, her ego was so identified with doing down dog a certain way that she wasn't able to break-through and work constructively.

Keeping the entire body strong, supple, and vibrant, is important even when an injury is present. A well-rounded, satisfying yoga practice that helps comforts the body and relaxes mind stay will help you deal with stress of having an injury. It is even more important to cultivate a physical and mental environment conducive to health and healing when you have an injury. In the case of this student, yoga may or may not have helped her with her shoulder. But, certainly, yoga would have helped her body and mind in every other way when she needed it most.

In addition to keeping the rest of the body and mind healthy while tending a shoulder injury, practicing yoga can make one feel more empowered and optimistic about recovery. This is an essential ballast against the sinking feeling of helplessness and fear that often accompany injuries. When one is actively involved in managing a difficult physical and/or emotional challenge there is a greater likelihood that their mind will stay focused and clear. Additionally, doing a modified yoga practice while you have an injury will help offset the negative association that one may have with the body. One may come to realize that the body is not a problem; rather, the body has a problem. By practicing yoga and recognizing everything that your body can do and everything that isn't wrong, one will have a much more positive perspective on one's physical reality.

The last major benefit of practicing yoga with an injury is that injuries provide us with greater self-awareness. Quite simply, injuries make us pay attention to our body. Very few people pause throughout their daily life to observe the sensations, actions, and other inner-workings of the body. But, there's nothing that will capture the mind and demand attention like a rotator cuff tear or frozen shoulder. While this isn't a pleasant experience, it does tend to foster a growth curve. We tend to prioritize learning more about our body and managing our well being when something is threatening our comfort and vitality. In this sense, short-term injuries can lead to greater long-term awareness and wellness strategies.

Appendix A:

Pre-surgical Checklist and Post Surgical instructions

Once the surgery is scheduled, you will receive the following checklist and instructions.

■ Pre-surgical instructions and Checklist:

- ❑ Confirm that you have noted your surgical date and check-in time.
- ❑ **You should have <u>no</u> food or drink (including gum, mints, etc.) starting the night before surgery.**
- ❑ Arrange transportation with a friend or family member to and from the surgical location. Directions are attached. (Allow sufficient travel time.)
- ❑ Pick up or receive your post-surgery medications prior to surgery. You should have your medication <u>BEFORE</u> your surgery date.
- ❑ You should have <u>no</u> food or drink (including gum, mints, etc.) starting the night before surgery.
- ❑ Stop the following medications at least seven days before surgery: Aspirin, Ibuprofen (Motrin, Advil), Naproxen (Aleve), Bextra, Vioxx, Celebrex.
- ❑ If you are on Coumadin/Warfarin, you should have received instructions from your doctor already. If not, contact the office.
- ❑ Take any high blood pressure medications on your regular schedule with a sip of water only.
- ❑ If you have Diabetes, Do not take any oral diabetic medication the morning of the surgery. If you inject insulin, use half of your normal dose the night before surgery. If there are any questions, speak with your medical doctor or call our office.
- ❑ Have a pre-surgery meeting with the physical therapist to discuss and prepare for your rehabilitation after surgery. You should have tentative dates planned for the start of the rehab after surgery.

<u>Post-Surgical Instructions</u>

The day of surgery, the nurses will go over the following information with you.

Post-Surgical Anesthesia Recovery

- ✓ You may feel dizzy, light-headed, or sleepy for the first twelve to twenty-four hours after your operation. **You cannot drive, operate any mechanical or electrical devices, drink alcohol, or make any important decisions for twenty-four hours and as long as you are taking prescribed narcotic medication.**
- ✓ If you have had general anesthesia, it is normal for you to feel generalized aching, sore muscles, and have a strange taste in your mouth, or possibly a sore throat. This is normal and will dissipate in twenty-four to forty-eight hours.
- ✓ If you had a regional anesthesia (interscalene block), your shoulder and arm may feel like it is asleep for up to eighteen hours after surgery. This is normal.
- ✓ Resume your diet gradually as tolerated.

Post-Surgical Pain Control: Medication and Ice

- ✓ Discomfort from the surgical site is normal and to be expected.
- ✓ You should have your pain medication BEFORE Surgery. If you do not, call the office and arrange for the medication. Start your pain medication once you get home even if you do not have pain. This ensures that your discomfort is at a low level. Usually, you should take the first pill when you get home.
- ✓ *Some patients after surgery have stomach sensitivity to pain medication. This can lead to nausea. Try and eat light food and drink before you start the medications, as this can help calm your stomach.*
- ✓ Ice therapy, with either ice bags or an ice unit, should be used for the first three to five days. This will keep swelling and pain diminished. Never put ice directly on the skin, and check regularly to make sure that the skin is not numb to the touch. If it is, remove the ice, allow the skin to warm up, and then reapply. If you have had a regional anesthetic your shoulder will be numb for up to 16hours. So you will have to remove the ice at regular intervals. Keep in mind that **you can give yourself frostbite, so you must use care; a general rule of thumb is twenty to thirty minutes on and twenty minutes rest from ice.**

Care of Dressing and Showering:

- ✓ In general, for arthroscopic surgery, you should keep the dressing on for twenty-four to forty-eight hours. There is usually a reddish watery drainage for the first day or so. This is normal. If there is actual bleeding soaking through, you should call your doctor.
- ✓ After forty-eight hours, you may remove the dressing along with the Band-Aids, and shower. After you shower, dry the area and cover incision sites with new dressings. **It is important to keep the incision sites clean, covered, and dry.**
- ✓ Report to the office any fever/chills, excessive swelling, redness to skin, yellow discolored drainage, uncontrolled pain, persistent nausea/vomiting, or any other concerns. Phones are attended to twenty-four hours a day.

Post-Op Visit

- ✓ The office will call you the next working day after surgery to let see k how you are doing and to confirm your follow-up appointment.

Sling and Exercises for Shoulder Arthroscopy

- ✓ **The sling is to be worn at all times, even to bed**. You may take the arm out only to do you pendulum exercises, internal and external rotation exercises, scapular exercises, and to perform your wrist and elbow exercises. You must do your exercises a minimum of three to five times every day.
- ✓ Formal Physical therapy will not start until your doctor instructs you that it is time to start.

Overview of Immediately after Surgery:
By Mena Brady, RN

When you start to wake up after surgery, you will be in the recovery area. This is called the PACU (post- anesthetic care unit). The nurse and anesthesiologist are there to help you wake up comfortably and safely. You will be attached to monitors for blood pressure, oxygen use, and temperature. These are referred to as your "vital signs." You will also have a tube (IV) for fluids and medicines in place usually in your hand or arm. This IV line is inserted before your surgery, in the pre-operative holding area. If you have had a regional anesthetic, your arm or leg may feel like it is asleep or numb. This regional anesthesia usually blocks any pain that surgery may have caused.

Once you are awake enough, your nurse will ask you questions about how you are feeling, specifically, if you are having any discomfort or pain. All healthcare facilities are now required to address patients' discomfort in a quantitative manner, that is, on a scale of zero to ten. You will be asked to rate your discomfort on this "Pain Scale." If you are having pain, you will receive medication to help lessen your pain. Some discomfort is common, but it is usually tolerable, and medicines are given to keep you comfortable. These medications may make you drowsier, but it is important to remember that you will be feeling sleepy and groggy for most of the day of surgery anyway. You have had anesthesia and it takes a while for it to clear from your system.

Do not make unrealistic plans for that day. It is a good idea to plan to go home and rest in bed, on the couch, or in a recliner for the rest of the day. You should arrange for someone to stay with you for at least the first twenty-four hours.

Some patients have nausea or vomiting after waking up from surgery. This may be related to anesthesia or post-operative pain medications. There are very good medicines that can be given to minimize any nausea and/or vomiting you may experience. So be sure to let the nurse know if you are experiencing any nausea.

Most patients are ready to go home within sixty to ninety minutes after arrival in the PACU. Patients often are sleepy and may have muscle aches. Other common symptoms are sore throat and occasional dizziness or headaches. These side effects after ambulatory anesthesia usually subside in the hours following surgery, but it may take several days before they are gone completely. Know that a period of recovery at home is common and to be expected. You will go home with either an ice pad or Ice bag to minimize swelling. Usually, you will go home with your arm in a sling. Often, patients take medication for after surgery *before* the surgery, as part of the preparation. It is important to take this medicine as ordered by your doctor. Always be sure to eat something before you take your pain medication. This will minimize the possible stomach upset from the medicines. Once pain starts and begins increasing, it is more difficult to get it under control. It is wise to begin taking your medicine as soon as you start to feel discomfort. You will be given written discharge instructions. These instructions will be reviewed with you and a responsible adult. This is because you may not fully understand or remember what is being said since you have received anesthetics and other medications. Be sure to look at these instructions from time to time after you get home. They will give you important information about your dressing, ice use/cold therapy, when to call the doctor, and other post-operative issues. Often you will chance your dressing at home one to two days after surgery. Taking a shower is usually okay, but should not be done till twenty four to forty-eight hours after surgery. The wound should be dried and re-dressed. Cold therapy via an ice unit, ice bag, or frozen peas is commonly used. This can help with the swelling and pain in the first three to five days. It is important to protect the skin from frostbite. A bandage or washcloth should be placed between the skin and the ice. You should check the skin every thirty to sixty minutes and ensure that it is not completely numb. However, if you have had a regional anesthesia, the skin will be numb already. As a protection, you should rest the skin from ice for twenty minutes every hour.

You will want to contact your doctor if:
- The pain or swelling (or both) continues or gets worse, or the pain is unrelieved by the pain medication;
- You notice redness or swelling, or if pus drains from the incision site;
- You have a fever higher than 101.5 F; or
- The incision site bleeds excessively.

Appendix B:

Home Therapy Exercise Prescription

Instructions:

1. Start exercises only when your surgeon directs you to do so. My patients are usually seen by the physical therapist BEFORE surgery to get their instructions.
2. Do the exercise sessions up to five times per day. Spread the sessions out over the day.
3. Don't lift any objects with your surgical arm during the first three weeks
4. Avoid forceful sudden or jerky movements.
5. It is best to space the exercise sessions out throughout the day (every two to three hours) to maintain flexibility during this important time of healing.
6. Do not use the surgical arm to push yourself out of bed or out of a chair during the first six weeks.
7. Do not do strengthening exercises until three months after surgery, unless otherwise instructed.

The following exercises have been prescribed by your physician (check all that apply).

Phase 1: Early Protected Motion:

❑ Exercise 1   Pendulum Exercise (Prehab)

❑ Exercise 2   Passive External Rotation with a Bar (Prehab)

❑ Exercise 3   Scapular Training (Prehab)

❑ Exercise 4   Elbow Flexion and Extension

❑ Exercise 5   Hand and Wrist Motion

Phase 2: Motion Recovery

❑ Exercise 6   Shoulder Flexion with Bar

❑ Exercise 7   Shoulder Flexion with Pulley

❑ Exercise 8   Shoulder Flexion Table Stretch

❑ Exercise 9   Wall Stretch for Posterior Shoulder

❑ Exercise 10   Internal Rotation with Pulley

❑ Exercise 11   External Rotation with Bar

Phase 3: Muscle Strengthening and Balance

❑ Exercise 12   External Rotation Strengthening

❑ Exercise 13   Internal Rotation Strengthening

❑ Exercise 14   Supraspinatus Strengthening

Exercise 1
Pendulum Exercise
(See Figure B-1)

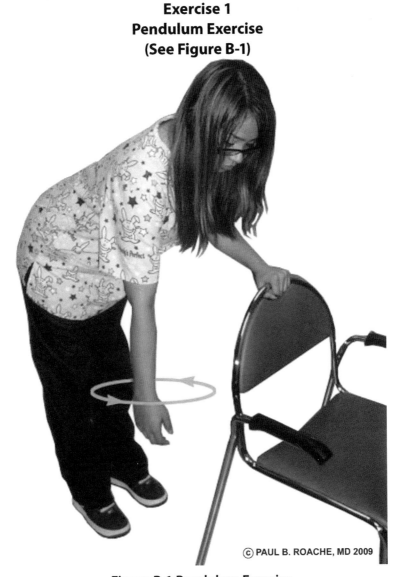

Figure B-1:Pendulum Exercise

1. Lean forward and use your unaffected arm to support you.
2. Let your surgical arm hang loosely.
3. Move your body and arm in a small, circular motion and gently swing the arm.
4. Note that it is the active motion of your body that causes the arm to move. You should not attempt to make the arm swing on its own.
5. Do this exercise for at least two minutes.

Exercise 2
Passive External Rotation with a Bar
(See Figures B-2 and B-3)

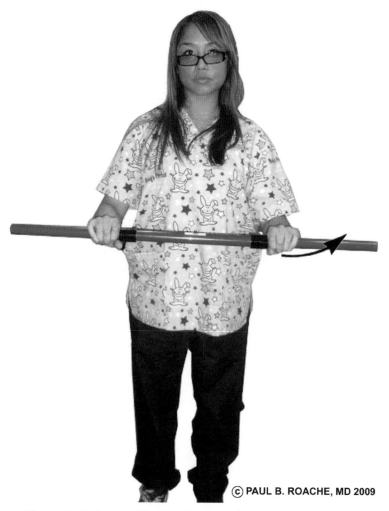

© PAUL B. ROACHE, MD 2009

Figure B-2: Start of Passive External Rotation with a Bar

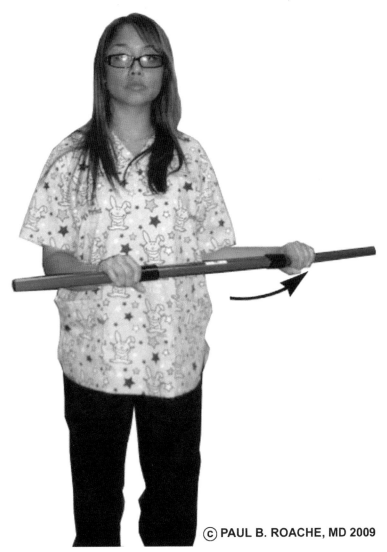

© PAUL B. ROACHE, MD 2009

Figure B-3: The finish of Passive External Rotation with a Bar

1. Stand or lie on your back on the floor.
2. Grasp the bar with both hands, with elbows against your body.
3. With the non-operative hand, move the bar toward the operative hand; this moves the hand away from the body.
4. Slowly perform ten repetitions.
5. Do this three to five times daily.

Exercise 3
Table Scapular Training
(See Figure B-4)

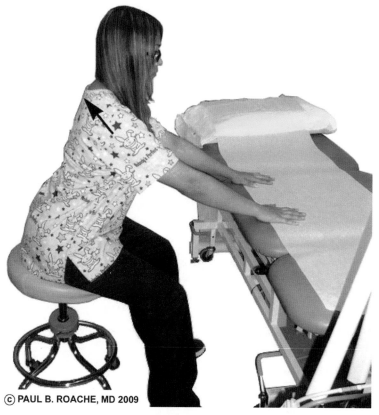

© PAUL B. ROACHE, MD 2009

Figure B-4: Table Scapular Training

1.   Sit on a chair or stool facing a table or desk.
2.   Place both hands flat on the table, with arms nearly straight, slightly wider than shoulder width.
3.   Pull both shoulder blades toward each other and hold for ten seconds.
4.   Release and repeat ten times. Perform three to five sets a day.

Exercise 4
Elbow Flexion and Extension
(See Figure B-5)

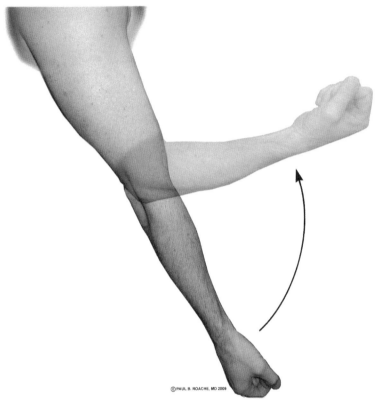

Figure B-5: Elbow Flexion and Extension

1. Keep your surgical shoulder stabilized while performing these exercises.
2. Straighten and bend your arm at the elbow.
3. Perform ten repetitions, five times per day for each exercise.
4. This can be performed while sitting or standing

Exercise 5
Hand and Wrist Motion
(See Figure B-6)

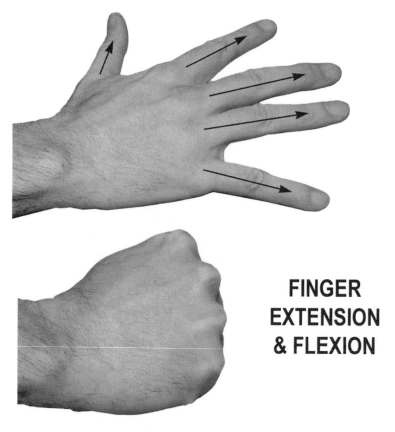

FINGER
EXTENSION
& FLEXION

© PAUL B. ROACHE, MD 2009

Figure B-6: Hand and Wrist Motion

1. Fully extend the fingers of your hand on the surgical side.
2. Squeeze your fingers together to make a fist.
3. Perform ten repetitions, five times per day for each exercise.
4. You can perform this exercise with the sling on or off.

Exercise 6
Shoulder Flexion with Bar
(See Figures B-7 and B-8)

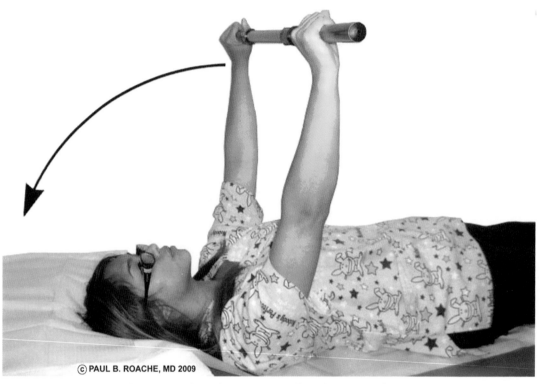

Figure B-7: Starting position for Flexion with Bar

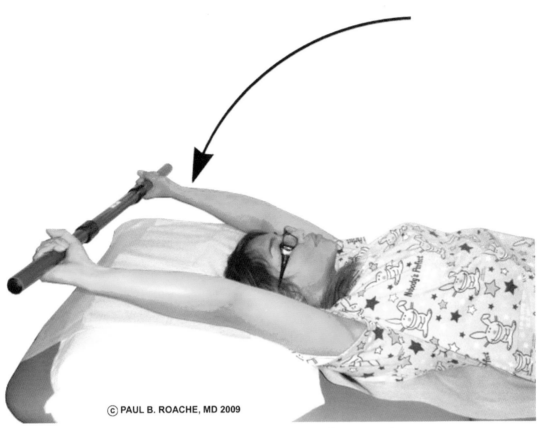

© PAUL B. ROACHE, MD 2009

Figure B-8: Finishing position for Flexion with Bar

1. Lie on your back as shown. Clasp your hands together or hold the bar with both hands as shown. (You do not need a bar to do this exercise, but if using a bar, place your hands close together.)
2. Raise both hands overhead so that you feel a stretch. Your surgical arm should be totally relaxed. Your range of motion should increase as each day passes.
3. Hold for thirty seconds. Increase to two minutes gradually over a few weeks.
4. Perform five to ten repetitions, five times per day (goal: 140° of elevation)

Exercise 7
Shoulder Flexion with Pulley
(See figures B-9 and B-10)

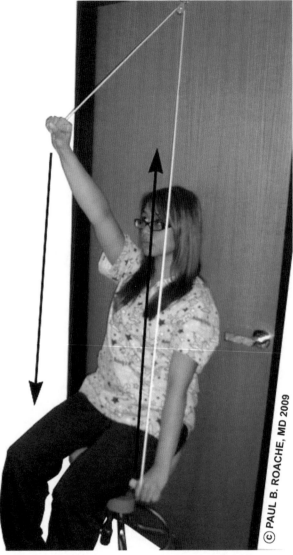

Figure B-9: Starting position for Flexion with Pulley

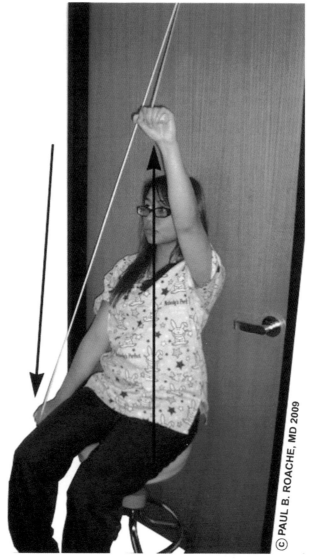

© PAUL B. ROACHE, MD 2009

Figure B-10: Finishing position for Flexion with Pulley

1. Sit in a chair with the pulley assembled as shown.
2. Raise the surgical arm overhead by pulling down on the pulley with the other hand so that you feel a stretch.
3. Hold thirty seconds and then slowly let gravity lower your surgical arm. Gradually work up to holding for two minutes over several weeks.
4. Perform five to ten repetitions, five times per day.
5. Do NOT use the surgical arm to lift the other arm.

Exercise 8
Shoulder Flexion Table Stretch
(See Figures B-11 and B-12)

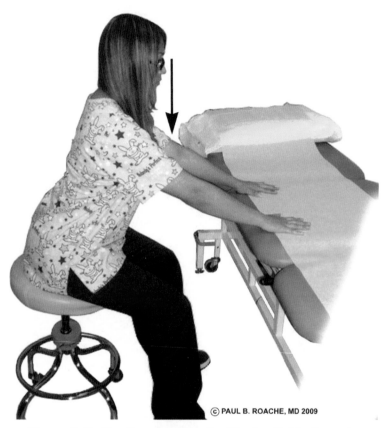

© PAUL B. ROACHE, MD 2009

Figure B-11: Starting position for Flexion Table Stretch

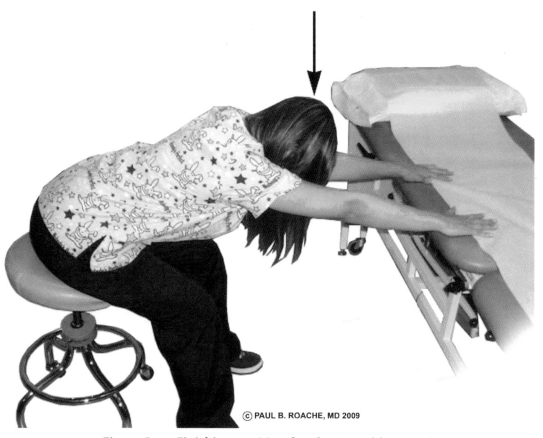

© PAUL B. ROACHE, MD 2009

Figure B-12: Finishing position for Flexion Table Stretch

1. Sit upright in a chair (preferably a chair with wheels).
2. Place both hands on a desktop or table in front of you.
3. Gently lean forward to stretch the shoulders. Keep shoulders square.
4. Hold for thirty seconds. Gradually work up to holding for two minutes over several weeks.
5. Perform five times daily.

Exercise 9
Wall Stretch for Posterior Shoulder
(See Figure B-13 and B-14)

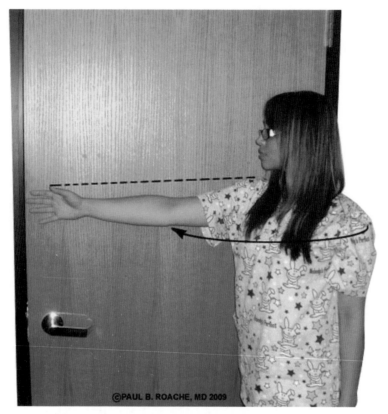

©PAUL B. ROACHE, MD 2009

Figure B-13: Starting position for Wall Stretch

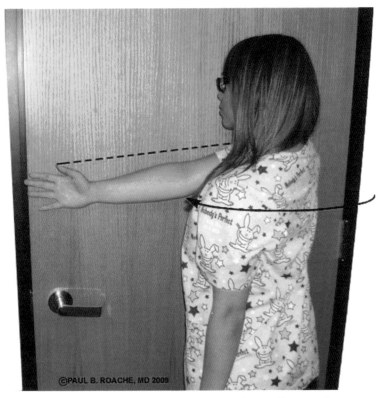

©PAUL B. ROACHE, MD 2009

Figure B-14: Finishing position for Wall Stretch

1. Stand with your shoulder against a wall or door.
2. Raise the arm to chest height. Try not to shrug the shoulder.
3. Keep the arm and shoulder against the wall; roll the body towards the arm.
4. Hold for thirty seconds. Gradually work up to holding for two minutes over several weeks.
5. Perform five times per day

Exercise 10
Internal Rotation with Pulley
(See Figures B-15 and B-16)

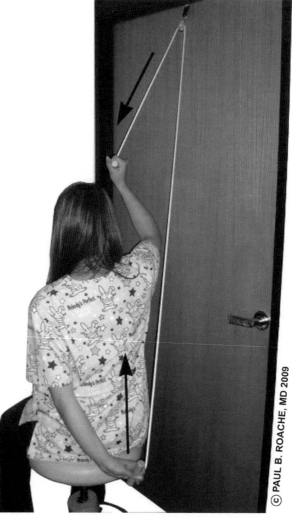

© PAUL B. ROACHE, MD 2009

Figure B-15: Starting position for Internal Rotation with Pulley

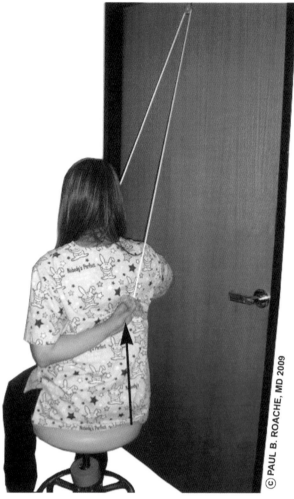

Figure B-16: Finishing position for Internal Rotation with Pulley

1. Hold pulley handle in operative hand behind your back with your arm straight.
2. Hold the other pulley handle above your head.
3. Push down on the upper handle and slowly raise the operative hand up your back.
4. When you reach a natural stopping point, hold for thirty seconds to two minutes.
5. Perform five to ten repetitions, five times a day.

Exercise 11
External Rotation with Bar
(See Figures B-17 and B-18)

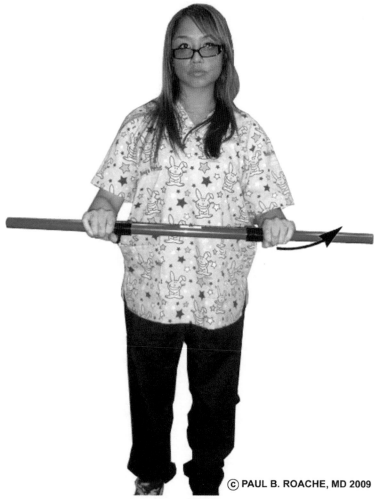

© PAUL B. ROACHE, MD 2009

Figure B-17: Starting position for External Rotation with Bar

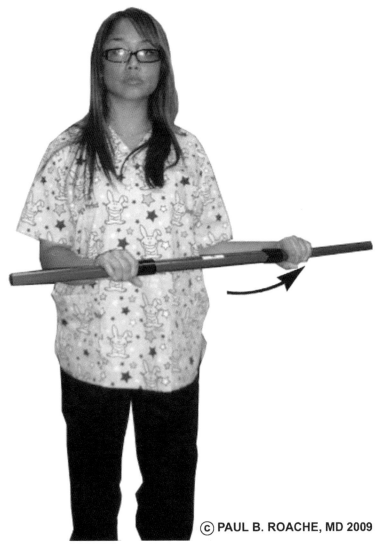

© PAUL B. ROACHE, MD 2009

Figure B-18: Finishing position for External Rotation with Bar

1. Stand or lie on your back with your elbows bent to 90° and hold a stick across your waist.
2. Using a stick for assistance, rotate your surgical arm and forearm away from your body to (circle one: 30°, 40°, 50°), BUT NO FURTHER.
3. Keep your elbows close to your sides at all times.
4. Hold ten to thirty seconds. Gradually increase to two minutes over several weeks.
5. Perform five to ten repetitions, five times per day.

Exercise 12
External Rotation Strengthening
(See Figures B-19 and B-20)

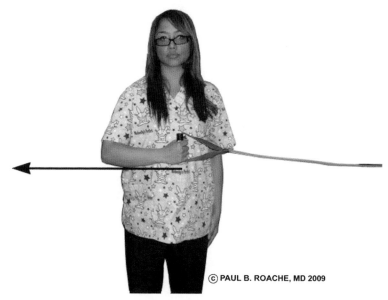

© PAUL B. ROACHE, MD 2009

Figure B-19: Starting position for External Rotation Strengthening

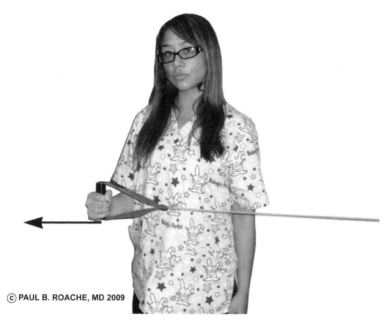

© PAUL B. ROACHE, MD 2009

Figure B-20: Finishing position for External Rotation Strengthening

1. Grab the handle of the stretch cord as shown, with the cord in front of your body.
2. Keeping your elbow at your side, move your hand outward away from your body.
3. Perform twenty to forty repetitions at slow to moderate pace, three times per day.

Exercise 13
Internal Rotation Strengthening
(See Figures B-21 and B-22)

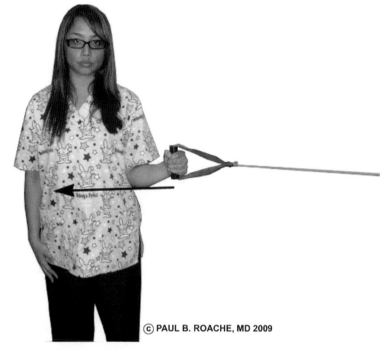

© PAUL B. ROACHE, MD 2009

Figure B-21: Starting position for Internal Rotation Strengthening

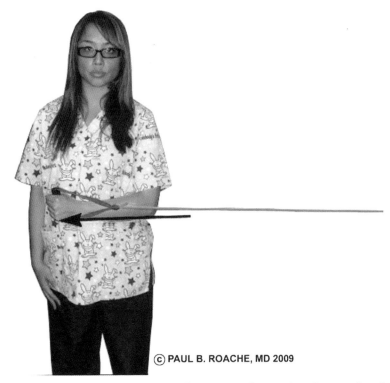

© PAUL B. ROACHE, MD 2009

Figure B-22: Finishing position for Internal Rotation Strengthening

1. Grab the handle of the stretch cord as shown, with the cord in front of your body.
2. Keeping your elbow at your side, move your hand inward toward your body.
3. Perform twenty to forty repetitions at slow to moderate pace, three times per day.

Exercise 14
Supraspinatus Strengthening
(See Figures B-23 and B-24)

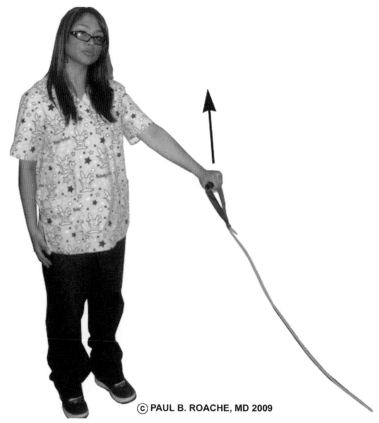

© PAUL B. ROACHE, MD 2009

Figure B-23: Starting position for Supraspinatus Strengthening

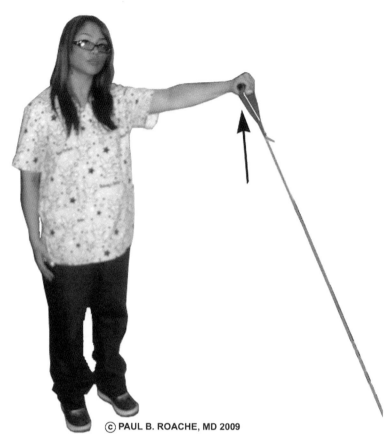

© PAUL B. ROACHE, MD 2009

Figure B-24: Finishing position for Supraspinatus Strengthening

1. Grab the handle of the stretch cord as shown, with the cord in front of your body and arm down and slightly out to the side, palm down.
2. Keeping your elbow at your side, move your hand upward toward shoulder height, but do not go above shoulder height.
3. Perform twenty to forty repetitions at slow to moderate pace, three times per day

Appendix C:

Guidelines for primary care physicians

How do you make the diagnosis?

These guidelines to confirm the diagnosis require matching the symptoms with the physical exam and understanding the treatments of the rotator cuff pathway.

If the answer to any of the following five questions is yes, then the patient has a high chance of having a rotator cuff injury and/or frozen shoulder.
Note: If dysfunction is from a fall or trauma, immediate X-ray and MRI is appropriate to detect an acute tear for surgical referral.

- Does the patient have pain from the shoulder at night that interrupts sleep?
- Does the patient have pain or difficulty while reaching above shoulder level?
- Are there any signs of rotator cuff weakness?
- Are there any signs of rotator cuff impingement?
- Are there any signs of loss of motion?

Rotator Cuff Weakness

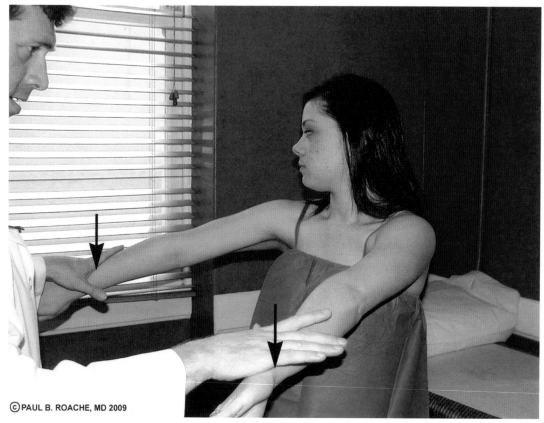

© PAUL B. ROACHE, MD 2009

Figure C-1: The Jobe Supraspinatus Test (JST)

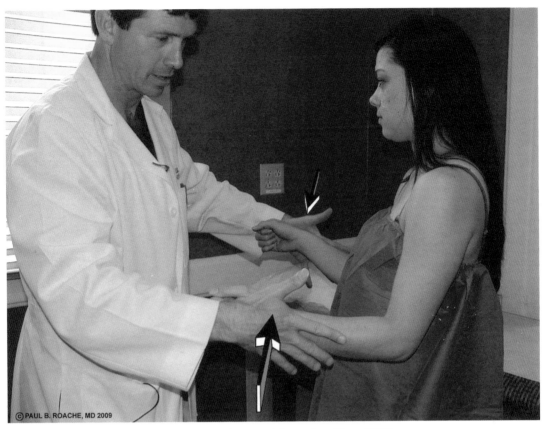

Figure C-2: External Rotation Test (ERT)

Impingement Signs

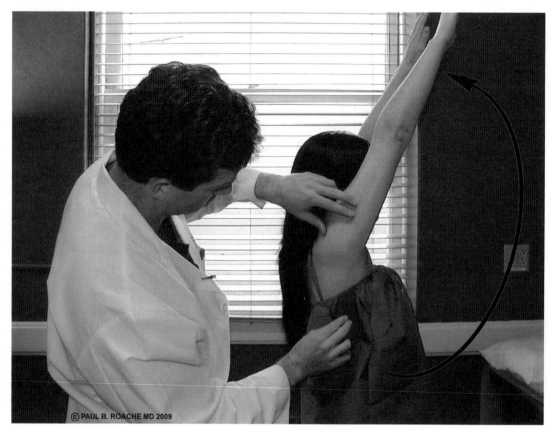

Figure C-3: Neer impingement sign

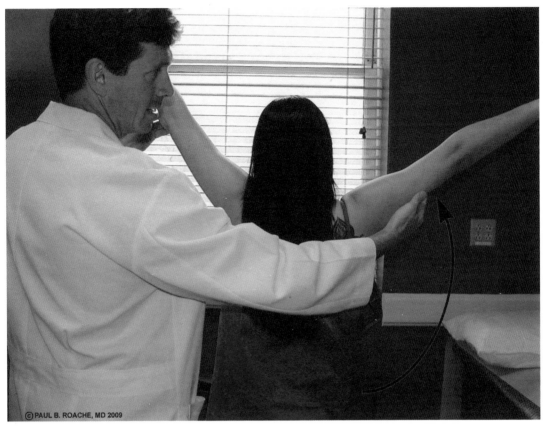

Figure C-4: Painful abduction arc sign

Motion Loss Testing

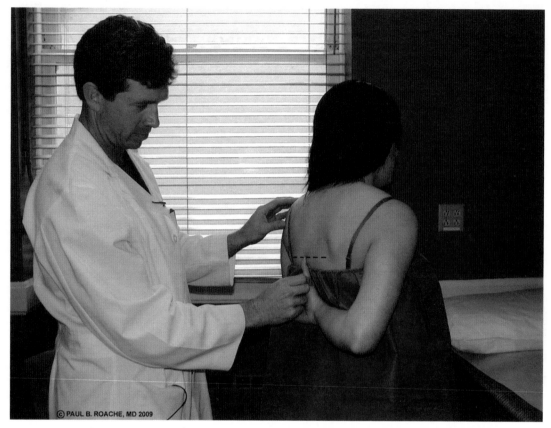

© PAUL B. ROACHE, MD 2009

Figure C-5: Internal rotation to the back (IRB or apley's scratch test):

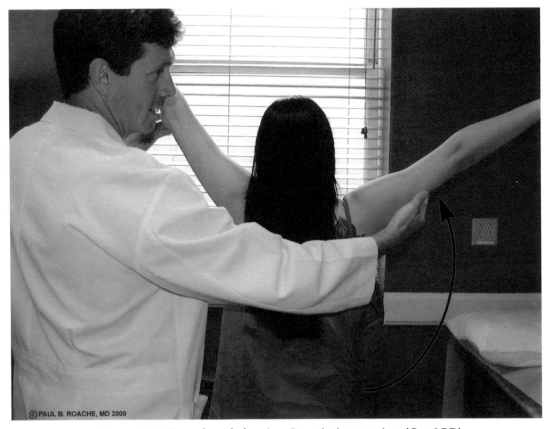

© PAUL B. ROACHE, MD 2009

Figure C-6: Capsular Abduction Restriction testing (CapABD)

When the history and examination indicate that there is a rotator cuff injury, and if initial treatments have been unsuccessful; it is time to reassess the diagnosis. A shoulder consultation for confirmation of the diagnosis and necessary injection(s) is valuable early in the injury process whether the patient is a surgical candidate or not. The correct diagnosis is essential for deciding upon proper treatment. This often requires a surgeon who is experienced in the history, examination, and imaging of the shoulder.

Consideration of X-rays, and MRI early in the evaluation will help confirm the diagnosis and identify rotator cuff tears that may need surgical repair.

6234997R1

Made in the USA
Charleston, SC
02 October 2010